Healing Words

ALSO BY LARRY DOSSEY, M.D.

Space, Time & Medicine
Beyond Illness
Recovering the Soul
Meaning and Medicine

HEALING
WORDS

THE POWER OF PRAYER AND
THE PRACTICE OF MEDICINE

LARRY DOSSEY, M.D.

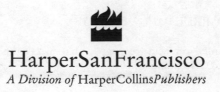

HarperSanFrancisco
A Division of HarperCollinsPublishers

HEALING WORDS: *The Power of Prayer and the Practice of Medicine.* Copyright © 1993 by Larry Dossey, M.D. All rights reserved. Printed in the United States of America. No part of this book may be used or reproduced in any manner whatsoever without written permission except in the case of brief quotations embodied in critical articles and reviews. For information address HarperCollins Publishers, 10 East 53rd Street, New York, NY 10022.

FIRST EDITION

Library of Congress Cataloging-in-Publication Data
Dossey, Larry. 1940–
    Healing words : the power of prayer and the practice of medicine /
Larry Dossey. — 1st ed.
      p. cm.
    Includes bibliographical references and index.
    ISBN 0–06–250251–4 (alk. paper). — ISBN 0–06–250252–2 (pbk. :
alk. paper)
    1. Healing—Religious aspects. 2. Prayer. I. Title.
BL65.M4D67   1993
291.4'3—dc20   92–56132
                                           CIP

94 95 96 97 ❖ RRD(H) 10 9 8 7 6 5

This edition is printed on acid-free paper that meets the American National Standards Institute Z39.48 Standard.

For Garry and Bet

Truly, it was to our amazement that the ailing said they were well. Being Europeans, we thought we had given away to doctors and priests our ability to heal. But here it was, still in our possession. . . . It was ours after all, we were more than we had thought we were.

—Alvar Nuñez Cabeza de Vaca to the king of Spain, early sixteenth century

Contents

Acknowledgments

To anyone contemplating writing a book on prayer, I advise having a saint around the house. It helps immensely. That is why my deepest gratitude is to Barbara, my wife.

I learned most about silence and solitude from my parents and grandparents, my earliest exemplars in prayer. I am deeply thankful to Kitty Farmer, who for years has lovingly labored in countless ways to disseminate my work, and to my literary agent, Muriel Nellis. I am grateful to Robert L. Martin, who provided the nudge I needed to begin this project; to Jeff Uffelman, brilliant Santa Fe artist and namer of books; to Tom Grady, Caroline Pincus, Robin Seaman, Clayton Carlson, Ani Chamichian, Jo Beaton, Terri Goff, Wendy Wells, and Kevin Bentley at HarperSanFrancisco, for their unstinting attention to detail.

To Juan and Rosa Ortega, I extend gratitude for almost three decades of lessons in unforced spirituality that have usually been demonstrated around campfires near timberline.

But there are more people to thank for the evolution of this book than I can possibly name. I offer a collective prayer of thanks to them all, and I hope they realize that this "nondirected approach" does not diminish my gratitude.

Author's Note

I have used a variety of terms throughout this book to refer to a Supreme Being. In most cases I have chosen as neutral a term as possible, such as the Absolute.

I tend to agree with those wise teachers who say that all the names of God are misleading. As all the major esoteric wisdom traditions tell us, the Absolute "cannot be spoken or thought." We simply have no reliable pictures of the Almighty. As the Sufi aphorism soberly states, "No man has seen God and lived."

In the fourteenth century, an anonymous English monk, believed to be the author of *The Cloud of Unknowing*, an exalted religious tract that deeply influenced the religious life of the time, added his lament to the futility of addressing and even thinking about the Universal. "But now you will ask me," said he, "'How am I to think of God himself, and what is he?' and I cannot answer you except to say 'I do not know!' For with this question you have brought me into the cloud of unknowing. [O]f God himself can no man think."[1]

As the great thirteenth-century German mystic Meister Eckhart observed, "Whoever perceives something in God and attaches thereby some name to him, that is not God. God is ineffable."[2] And, "It is God's nature to be without a nature."[3]

At this moment in history, in which we're experiencing a much-needed awakening of feminine values, perhaps it is important to point out that the problem of naming the Absolute is not resolved merely by replacing all the masculine names and pronouns with feminine ones. "God" and "Goddess," he and she, founder equally. The Absolute is radically beyond any description whatsoever, including gender.

With these limitations in mind, the reader may insert, in every instance that follows, his or her preferred name for the Absolute—whether Goddess, God, Allah, Krishna, Brahman, the Tao, the Universal Mind, the Almighty, Alpha and Omega, the One.

Preface

A few years ago, I was surprised to discover a single scientific study that strongly supported the power of prayer in getting well. Because I'd never heard of controlled experiments affirming prayer, I assumed this study stood alone. But did it? Somehow I could not let the matter rest, and I began to probe the scientific literature for further proof of prayer's efficacy. I found an enormous body of evidence: over one hundred experiments exhibiting the criteria of "good science," many conducted under stringent laboratory conditions, over half of which showed that prayer brings about significant changes in a variety of living beings.

I was astonished. I had begun my search believing it would turn up little. After all, if scientific proof for the healing effects of prayer existed, surely it would be common knowledge among scientifically trained physicians. I came to realize the truth of what many historians of science have described: A body of knowledge that does not fit with prevailing ideas can be ignored as if it does not exist, no matter how scientifically valid it may be. Scientists, including physicians, can have blind spots in their vision. The power of prayer, it seemed, was an example.

The question I *then* had to deal with made me very uncomfortable: What was I personally going to *do* with this information? Would I ignore it, or allow it to affect the way I practiced medicine? These uncertainties distilled to a single question from which I could not escape: *Are you going to pray for your patients or not?*

For many years I'd ignored prayer. I considered it an arbitrary, optional frill that simply was not in the same league as drugs and surgery. I had in fact tried to *escape* spiritual or religious influences in healing, fancying myself a *scientific* physician.

I grew up in a world that no longer exists—the sharecropper, cotton-growing culture of central Texas. Prayer and Protestantism permeated those bleak prairies and, with few exceptions, everyone living on them. The one-room country church, situated forlornly amid cotton fields at a crossroads, was the hub around which life revolved. Alongside the church was the "tabernacle," a shingle-roofed, open-air structure used in the steamy, sultry summers for outdoor revival meetings. People gathered at the church twice on Sunday and on Wednesday nights to sing, pray, testify, and hear the preacher—usually a young ministerial student from Baylor University in nearby Waco—spew forth sermons flavored with hideous and terrifying descriptions of hellfire, damnation, and eternal punishment (sermons about heaven were far less frequent).

As a child I never doubted the truth of what I heard. I took it all seriously. By age fourteen I was the pianist for the tiny church and an eager participant in "youth revivals." By age sixteen I was touring as pianist with a traveling gospel quartet, and I played gospel piano as well for an itinerant tent evangelist known all over the state for his fiery earnestness. I planned to become a minister, but aborted at the last moment my plans to attend Baylor University, the world's largest Baptist school. My twin brother, who is today a retired dentist and a nature mystic, was for some reason blessedly unaffected by all this religious fervor and took a nonchalant attitude toward it. When it came time to leave the farm for college, he convinced me that the wiser course was to enroll in "the University"—of Texas, in Austin. Looking back, there were strong omens that this was the right choice. By the time we left for college, the frail, one-room church had begun to lean precariously toward the south, as if pointing the way toward Austin. The tabernacle was actually falling down; the gospel quartet had broken up; and the tent evangelist had been killed in a plane crash.

The university proved my religious undoing. Protestant fundamentalists have always had trouble with scientific materialism, and I was no exception. Under its withering influence, and aided by my discovery of Bertrand Russell, Aldous Huxley, and other intellectual giants, my religious fervor wilted like a central Texas cotton field in September. I became an agnostic.

Medical school followed college, then a stint in the Army as a battalion surgeon in Vietnam. By the time I eventually finished my training in internal medicine and began private practice, I had begun to regrow my spiritual roots. A major event in this process was my discovery during medical school of the philosophies of the East, particularly Buddhism and Taoism. I read widely and insatiably the works of Eastern mystics and Western commentators. I was delightfully surprised to discover that their core teachings were not just Eastern but universal, appearing also in the esoteric traditions of the major Western spiritual traditions. I found that Western mysticism has periodically been just as vibrant as in the East, although not as well known. Feeling the need for a practice in addition to a philosophy, I began to meditate. This was somewhat difficult in Texas in those days. Unlike now, there were scarcely any meditation instructors, teachers, or gurus, and "meditation" was still a dirty word. But a few wise books on meditative practice had just begun to emerge, and I put their instructions to good use. With immense difficulty and struggle, I gradually adopted an eclectic philosophy that was more spiritually satisfying than anything I had grown up with.

Even so, the experimental data on prayer that I turned up caught me off guard. I really wanted nothing to do with it. Meditation was acceptable, but the thought of "talking to God" in prayer was reminiscent of the fundamental Protestantism I felt I had laid to rest. Yet the results of the prayer experiments kept forcing themselves into my psyche.

These studies showed clearly that prayer can take many forms. Results occurred not only when people prayed for explicit outcomes, but also when they prayed for nothing specific. Some studies, in fact, showed that a simple "Thy will be done" approach was quantitatively more powerful than when specific results were held in the mind. In many experiments, a simple attitude of prayerful*ness*—an all-pervading sense of holiness and a feeling of empathy, caring, and compassion for the entity in need—seemed to set the stage for healing.

Experiments with people showed that prayer positively affected high blood pressure, wounds, heart attacks, headaches, and anxiety.

The subjects in these studies also included water, enzymes, bacteria, fungi, yeast, red blood cells, cancer cells, pacemaker cells, seeds, plants, algae, moth larvae, mice, and chicks; and among the processes that had been influenced were the activity of enzymes, the growth rates of leukemic white blood cells, mutation rates of bacteria, germination and growth rates of various seeds, the firing rate of pacemaker cells, healing rates of wounds, the size of goiters and tumors, the time required to awaken from anesthesia, autonomic effects such as electrodermal activity of the skin, rates of hemolysis of red blood cells, and hemoglobin levels.[1]

Remarkably the effects of prayer did not depend on whether the praying person was in the presence of the organism being prayed for, or whether he or she was far away; healing could take place either on site or at a distance. Nothing seemed capable of stopping or blocking prayer. Even when an "object" was placed in a lead-lined room or in a cage that shielded it from all known forms of electromagnetic energy, the effect still got through.

These experiments prompted me to continue saying to myself: "The evidence seems to show that prayer works. You claim to be a scientific doctor. Are you going to follow these scientific directions and actually *use* prayer?"

Over time I decided that *not* to employ prayer with my patients was the equivalent of deliberately withholding a potent drug or surgical procedure. I felt I should be true to the traditions of scientific medicine, which means going *through* scientific data and not *around* it, no matter how uncomfortable it might be to do so and no matter how it might shake up one's favored beliefs. I simply could not ignore the evidence for prayer's effectiveness without feeling like a traitor to the scientific tradition. And so, after weighing these factors for many months, I concluded that I would pray for my patients. But how? I felt I could not pray the way I'd learned as a child. The old images of prayer I had grown up with—pleading with an elderly, robed, bearded, white male figure who preferred English—were hopelessly unsatisfying. As a child I'd made endless lists of everyone I could think of who was needy, which I obsessively and joylessly recited to the Almighty almost daily. I'd taken great pains to specify all the desired outcomes, having been taught that this was "the" way to pray. But this no longer felt right, so I invented a prayer ritual that seemed to square with my current spiritual inclinations and beliefs. I would go to my office earlier than usual each morning, ceremoniously light incense, and enter a prayerful, meditative frame of mind. As the incense filled the room, I would invoke the Absolute, asking only that "Thy will be done" in the lives of the patients I was about to see on early-morning hospital rounds, as well as those patients I would encounter that day in the office. For reasons I shall discuss later, never once did I pray for specific outcomes—for cancers to go away, for heart attacks to be healed, for diabetes to vanish. "May the best possible outcome prevail" was the strategy I preferred, not specifying what "best" meant.

I did not actually encourage my patients to pray. I didn't have to. This was Texas, which almost certainly meant that they would be praying vigorously, and that they would already be on more prayer lists than I could count. I enjoyed knowing this was a collaborative effort, and that we didn't have to talk about it. This suited my personal preferences for privacy in spiritual matters, and was compatible with my abhorrence of religious evangelism.

As part of the ritual I devised, I would shake several rattles and gourds, paraphernalia used worldwide by shamans and healers to "invoke the powers." These curious objects had been given to me by patients and friends over the years. When I used them, I felt a connection with healers of all cultures and ages. Although I had never imagined that I—a white-coated, scientifically trained modern doctor—would be behaving like this, my prayer ritual was deeply satisfying.

One morning things took an unexpected turn. In my enthusiasm I lit too much incense and set off the smoke alarm in my office. I was paid a sudden visit by the fire inspector of the hospital, who was quite irate about "that funny smell." I was not deterred, however, and I continued to pray for my patients until I left the actual practice of internal medicine five years ago. Did prayer make a difference? Was I a better doctor as a result of it? I do not know. I did no controlled, scientific, before-and-after studies to find out. I believe the answer is yes, however, if for no other reason than that I felt more connected with those I served.

My resistance to using prayer in my medical practice was not unique. Almost all scientifically oriented physicians experience it. It simply is difficult to retain a spiritual instinct if one travels the path of science. The message of modern medical education is clear: one must choose either logical, analytical, and rational approaches, or irrational, religious, superstitious, and "right-brained" ones, which include prayer. But the choice between science and spirituality appears increasingly artificial today, even from a scientific perspective. It is now possible to tell a new story, one that allows science and spirituality to stand side by side in a complementary way, neither trying to usurp or eliminate the other.[2]

Over the years I have often wondered why so few of my patients have discussed with me their religious feelings and prayers during their own illness or the illnesses of their loved ones. I can think of at least three possible reasons. First, few may actually have prayed or applied their religion to the problem at hand, so there was nothing to discuss. This seems unlikely. I practiced medicine in the Bible Belt—in the *buckle* of the Bible Belt, some said—where religiosity is endemic and a lot of praying goes on all the time. Second, they may have thought I would disapprove or think poorly of their religious views and their praying. Neither does this seem to hold. I had written several books about the role of consciousness and spiritual factors in health and illness, which many of my patients had read. They knew of my openness to these issues and that I would discuss them if asked. The third possibility seems most reasonable: they simply wanted these issues to remain private.

I have come to believe that patients do not wish, by and large, to bring their religion into their relationship with their physician. Something about mixing religion and the practice of medicine seems as odious and dangerous as letting church and state mingle. The task of the physician is to render medical expertise and emotional and psychological support to those we serve. Patients who want more may ask us to become involved at deeper levels; but it is best that they, not the doctor, take the initiative.

Not every physician agrees. Following a year as a battalion surgeon in Vietnam, I was assigned as a general medical officer to Fort Carson in Colorado Springs, Colorado. I served in the same clinic with two civilian doctors hired by the Army to care for the large numbers of military dependents in the area. These two physicians were "born-again" Christians and deeply religious. The first thing a patient saw on being seated in their office was the Bible, prominently displayed along-side medical books and journals. It was widely known that they used Christian principles in their medical practice, and many patients flocked to them for this reason. But there was another side: other patients, who wanted their medical care untinged by the personal religious views of their doctor, refused to consult them.

Also, for a brief period in my early days of private practice, I was on the staff of a hospital in which two psychiatrists practiced "Christian psychiatry." They were extremely vocal about this and were quite pop-ular locally.

These two experiences troubled me. I believe that physicians should not use their medical authority as a platform for espousing their private religious beliefs. Patients, particularly when severely ill, are often terribly vulnerable to anything a physician suggests, which makes it all too easy for physicians to prey on them in the name of their per-sonal religious credo. Quite simply, it is a shameful abuse of power. I therefore want to make it clear that I am not "selling" prayer in this book. I want only to discuss what in my opinion is a neglected area of medical science, for patients to do with as they wish.

I emphatically do not believe that physicians should impose their spiritual beliefs on their patients. For the physician who feels the need to do something that goes beyond physical means, however, prayer is perhaps the best method. Because the scientific evidence strongly sug-gests that prayer works nonlocally, or at a distance, physicians may pray privately for those they serve. This would spare patients all the homilies and easy answers that all too often are offered to the susceptible sick in the name of religion. And patients who want more may ask for it. When they do, it is wise to ask a third party, perhaps a member of the clergy, to become involved. After all, we do not allow priests and minis-ters and rabbis to perform appendectomies; neither should we expect physicians to regulate the spiritual lives of their patients, as if a white coat, stethoscope, or scalpel conferred on them some special spiritual expertise.

Many of the clinical cases that follow are taken from the author's practice of internal medicine. The names of all patients have been changed to preserve confidentiality.

Introduction

> Wherever there are no limits, where Infinity and Eternity
> and Immortality exist, that is where God is.
>
> —Mikhael Aivanhov, *The Mystery of Light*

   In spite of an obvious and widespread enthusiasm for prayer among Americans,[1] even the few researchers and critics who are cordial to investigating prayer scientifically feel that there is little hard evidence to support its effectiveness in healing. Stanley Krippner, director of Graduate Studies at San Francisco's Saybrook Institute, and one of the most authoritative investigators of the variety of unorthodox healing methods used around the world, has recently stated,

> From a critical view we would conclude that the research data on distant, prayer-based healing are promising, but too sparse to allow any firm conclusion to be drawn. . . . [I]f the effect is a strong one, it should be replicable by other investigators, but to date, research data on distant healing have not yielded a pattern of replicability. . . . Nevertheless, it is encouraging to observe that a beginning has been made to explore these types of reported effects as the implications for healing are profound.[2]

Psychologist Lawrence LeShan has studied distant healing perhaps more thoroughly than anyone. He has been struck by the paradoxes of this area, including the fact that miracles and failures seem frequently to stand side by side. LeShan emphasizes a remark by George Bernard Shaw that Lourdes is the most blasphemous place on the face of the earth: mountains of wheelchairs and piles of crutches exist, "but not a single wooden leg, glass eye, or toupée!" This is evidence, Shaw maintained, that God's power is limited; there are things he apparently cannot do, and this is blasphemy.[3]

For decades LeShan studied psychic healers, most of whom used some type of prayerful intervention in their work. He actually became a healer himself and taught these techniques to more than four hundred people. Writing in the late 1980s, he offered, like Krippner, a rather desultory summary of his experience:

> In all the many hundreds of healing encounters I and the people in the training groups participated in, there was never developed any ability to tell in advance which ones would result in medically unexpected biological changes, and which would not. We observed these changes taking place shortly after the healings quite often (my best estimate is about 15 to 20 percent of the time), but could never predict in advance any specific healing.[4]

This is far from heartening. If a drug or surgical procedure worked haphazardly and was effective only 20 percent of the time at best, it would never be approved and adopted into medical use but dismissed as practically worthless, and the search would continue for a better therapy.

If Krippner and LeShan are correct—as I believe they are—why focus on the role of prayer in healing? As I contemplated writing this book, I asked myself this question many times.

The most practical reason to examine prayer in healing is simply that, at least some of the time, *it works.* The evidence is simply overwhelming that prayer functions at a distance to change physical processes in a variety of organisms, from bacteria to humans. These data, which we will later examine, are so impressive that I have come to regard them as among the best-kept secrets in medical science.

The most important reason for examining the effects of prayer, however, has little to do with its healing effects in illness. The fact that prayer works says something incalculably important about our nature, and how we may be connected with the Absolute. We shall examine these implications shortly.

But what of the fact that prayer, overall, is not as effective as we might wish—a maximum of 20 percent, LeShan believes, even in the best of hands? This should be seen in a particular perspective. According to healers who routinely employ prayer, it is more effective for some problems than others. This should not be surprising. Penicillin is a miracle drug for strep throat, but is worthless for tuberculosis. If the effectiveness of penicillin were judged by applying it to all known infections, it would likely be effective far *less* than 20 percent of the time. But this would be an unfair assessment of penicillin. Therapies should be judged according to their effects in conditions in which they work, and prayer is no exception.

Some might argue that the analogy between prayer and penicillin is off base. If prayer represents the power of the Absolute, as George Bernard Shaw implied, then it should be effective in *all* diseases. But prayer involves more than the power of the Almighty; it is set in motion by human beings, who may be the weak link in an otherwise immensely strong chain. The fact that prayer doesn't work as powerfully and predictably as it might, therefore, may reflect deficiencies not of prayer, but of the pray-er.

Almost anyone can find in their own experience evidence of this possibility. Growing up in Texas, I was continually astonished by the bizarre ways people used prayer. In autumn hundreds of cities and towns all over the state would passionately engage in the Friday night ritual of high school football. As part of the pregame ceremony, opposing teams would gather in their respective locker rooms and huddle for the team prayer, in which the earnest young gladiators would pray to the same God for victory and for help in reducing their opponents to smithereens. How could both team's prayers possibly be answered?

This perverse use of prayer is not, of course, confined to football-crazed Texans. Prayers by opposing teams for victory are universal. Most recently, in the Persian Gulf war, Americans prayed to God for aid in defeating Iraq, while the Iraqis were simultaneously beseeching Allah to exterminate the Western infidels. What's a God to do?

It is difficult, of course, for combatants *not* to pray for victory, and it is difficult for sick and dying people not to pray for victory over their illness. I share these feelings. As a physician I would dearly love to have a magic bullet—a miracle drug or surgical procedure or prayer—that never failed when my patients needed it. But it is not difficult to imagine how a 100 percent success rate for prayer would create unimaginable global havoc. If all prayers for recovery during sickness were uniformly answered, almost no one would die—in which case our planet's population would have skyrocketed millennia ago and rendered our Earth unfit for human habitation. Even in situations that seem straightforward, an answered prayer may be cruelty in disguise, a blight against our existence. Oscar Wilde's aphorism applies: "When the gods want to punish us, they answer our prayers." Or as C. S. Lewis once wrote, "If God had granted all the silly prayers I've made in my life, where should I be now?"[5]

These observations may seem hopelessly abstract and of no comfort when we are ill, but we need to realize that the greater good for humankind, as well as for the planet, may be incompatible with the survival of every human who becomes sick. The fact that we invariably prefer prayer to eradicate illness suggests, unfortunately, that *we are not wise enough to use a prayer that works 100 percent of the time.* In view of our limitations, perhaps the wisest course for a caring, benevolent Supreme Being would be to curb the effects of prayers and ignore many if not most of them. Placing limits on the power of prayer would be a finite blessing, a gift in disguise. This would reduce its danger to us, and our danger to ourselves.

It would also be confusing—for we would see tantalizing, *occasional* examples of prayer's power, but *never* would we see prayer working reliably, all the time. This would mean that *there would be no formula*, no perfect way to pray, that humans could follow to produce a powerful and predictable result in all situations. It would thus appear that the Supreme Being had "scrambled" prayer—destroyed all the codes, abolished all the formulas—*anything* to prevent an invariable effect of prayer when used by inept, unwise beings.

If there actually were a built-in limitation to the manifest power of prayer, what would the resulting situation look like? It might mean that the effects of prayer would sometimes seem miraculous and at other times nonexistent. We would be unable to "catch" prayer in laboratory experiments as often as we wish. Even when these effects were statistically significant, they would seldom be smashingly dramatic. As a result, incessant debates would flow back and forth between prayer enthusiasts and critics. Titanic efforts would be made by skeptics to explain away any possible effect of prayer. Because some investigators would be able to tease out the effect of prayer more often than others, critics would argue that this capriciousness is evidence that prayer does not really work. Theologians would invent ingenious, convoluted defenses to prop up prayer and explain why it works only part of the time. Just when the skeptics seemed to be getting the upper hand in this endless debate, the "occasional miracle" would erupt or a new prayer study would surface, adding fuel to the fire. Laypeople, less concerned with the haggling between scientists and clerics than with prayer's occasional successes, would continue to believe in prayer and pray as usual. They would not be holding their breath awaiting the results of the latest double-blind, controlled experiment. Sound familiar? This scenario, which currently exists, may be evidence that the Universal Intelligence has indeed limited the power of prayer—for our own good.

WHAT IS PRAYER?

What *is* prayer? "Prayer" comes from the Latin *precarius*, "obtained by begging," and *precari*, "to entreat"—to ask earnestly, beseech, implore. This suggests two of the commonest forms of prayer—*petition*, asking something for one's self, and *intercession*, asking something for others. There also are prayers of *confession*, the repentance of wrongdoing and the asking of forgiveness; *lamentation*, crying in distress and asking for vindication; *adoration*, giving honor and praise; *invocation*, summoning the presence of the Almighty; and *thanksgiving*, offering gratitude. But like the 108 names for the Ganges in Hinduism, the classification of prayer can seem endless; theologian Richard J. Foster describes twenty-one separate categories.[6]

The complex ways in which prayer manifests in the human psyche have been eloquently described by theologian Ann Ulanov and Professor Barry Ulanov. Prayer, they state, is the most fundamental, primordial, and important "language" humans speak—"primary speech," they call it. "Prayer starts without words and often ends without them," they say. "It knows its own evasions, its own infinite variety of dodges. It works some of the time in signs and symbols, lurches when it must, leaps when it can, has several kinds of logic at its disposal. . . . "[7]

Prayer may be individual or communal, private or public. It may be offered in words, sighs, gestures, or silence.[8] Prayer may be a conscious activity, of course, but as we shall see, it may flow also from the depths of the unconscious. Prayer may even emerge in dreams, completely bypassing our waking awareness.

In researching the role of prayer in healing, I was surprised that so many authorities on prayer failed to define it in their books and papers on the subject. Now I think I know why. If prayer has its roots in the unconscious, we can never fully grasp its nature. This means that a complete definition of prayer can never be given.

The primary reason to focus on the role of prayer in healing is not to prove its effectiveness scientifically—although this can be done, I feel, and is one of the tasks of this book. The best reason goes deeper: *Prayer says something incalculably important about who we are and what our destiny may be.* As we shall see, prayer is a genuinely *nonlocal* event—that is, it is not confined to a specific place in space or to a specific moment in time. Prayer reaches outside the here-and-now; it operates at a distance and outside the present moment. Since prayer is initiated by a mental action, this implies that there is some aspect of our psyche that also is genuinely nonlocal. If so, then something of ourselves is infinite in space and time—thus omnipresent, eternal, and immortal. "Nonlocal," after all, does not mean "really big" or "a very long time." It implies *infinitude* in space and time, because a limited nonlocality is a contradiction in terms. In the West this infinite aspect of the psyche has been referred to as the soul. Empirical evidence for prayer's power, then, is indirect evidence for the soul. It is also evidence for shared qualities with the Divine—"the Divine within"—since infinitude, omnipresence, and eternality are qualities that we have attributed also to the Absolute.

The fact that we are capable of engaging in a nonlocal activity such as prayer has stunning spiritual implications. These dwarf the practical, immediate concerns about prayer, such as whether it can bail us out of difficulty when we need it.

The way prayer is conceived by most Western religions is far different from this: God is installed outside us, usually high above, as if in stationary orbit, functioning as a sort of master communications satellite. We "send" our prayers "upward" to God, who may or may not choose to function as a relay station to the object of our prayer. This scenario, with God up there and us down here, allows us to maintain a quite local version of who we are—isolated creatures of the moment locked in a linear, flowing time, confined to the body and awaiting death, ultimately sinful and unworthy, and whose only hope is to be redeemed by the merciful act of a Supreme Being. Although this vision may be comforting for millions of people—those who are convinced they are "saved" or "chosen," or who belong to some religious in-group—it causes immense confusion and guilt for others, and has been the source of untold nastiness in human affairs throughout recorded history. When compared with other religious views worldwide, this exteriorization of God and the resulting devaluation of humankind's innate nature appears to be, according to the late mythologist Joseph Campbell, a uniquely "pathological mythology."

Many people believe that the nature of prayer has already been adequately defined by the major Western religions, and that tampering with these age-old concepts is akin to heresy. Yet there is a case to be made for a dynamic, changing view. As Joseph Campbell once said, if a mythology does not continue to evolve, it dies. Those who believe that our understanding of prayer is essentially complete and should not continually be reevaluated may unwittingly be condemning prayer to death.

The old biblically based views of prayer, which are still largely in vogue, were developed when a view of the world was in place that is now antiquated and incomplete. In this century our fundamental ideas about how the universe works have changed. We have redefined our ideas about the nature of space, time, energy, and causation. These bear little resemblance to the views that dominated human thought for millennia in the West, and that shaped our concepts of prayer. In addition, our basic ideas of the structure and function of the human psyche have been radically transformed and continue to evolve. If our world view has changed, perhaps we should also reevaluate our views of the nature of prayer.

If the traditional, biblical, Western views of prayer were updated to a "modern" model, we could make the comparisons shown in Table 1, and elaborated throughout this book:

TABLE 1 **Models of Prayer**

	TRADITIONAL WESTERN MODEL	"MODERN" MODEL
Energy characteristic	"Energy" of some sort is "sent" to the "object" of prayer.	No actual energy is sent; "information" may be better term than "energy."
Temporal characteristic	Prayer is offered in the present: the goal is to affect the present or future events that have not yet happened.	Prayer effects are not confined to the present or future; they may also affect past events even though they seem already to have taken place—"time-displaced prayer."
Spatial characteristic	Prayer is "sent" elsewhere, usually to a Supreme Being who is "out there." This external entity then relays the prayer to its object—God as communications satellite.	There is no place for prayer to go because it is inherently "nonlocal"—i.e., it is infinite in both space and time. Moreover, if "the kingdom of Heaven is within"—the "Divine within" concept that is a part of most of the world's religious traditions—one cannot in principle pray to an entity outside one's Self.
Relationship to the Absolute	An external God is a necessary intermediary for prayer to work.	An external God is not regarded as a necessary intermediary because if nothing is "sent," then there is nothing to mediate; and if God is present to some degree in all individuals, the Divine factor in prayer is internal, not external, to everyone.
Source of origin in the psyche	Originates in conscious "waking" awareness. Prayer must be "thought," "contemplated," or somehow expressed consciously.	Originates either in conscious awareness or the unconscious part of the psyche. Prayer need not always be "thought"; "unconscious prayer"—even "dream prayer"—is thus possible.*

*At this point, I offer this "modern" model of prayer only tentatively; it will be explained and elaborated throughout the book.

TESTING PRAYER IN THE LAB

My belief that prayer can and should be tested experimentally has resulted in large measure from my experience as a physician. It is simply a fact that patients sometimes improve dramatically following prayer; and in my judgment, when something affects human bodies, it becomes the legitimate concern of medicine to find out more about it—scientifically, if possible—by asking certain questions. Among them:

• Was the patient's improvement a result of the prayer, or was it a chance correlation and a mere coincidence?

• If prayer actually caused the improvement, how did it do so?

• How reliable is prayer?

• If prayer does work, is it potent enough to be used alone, or should it be combined with orthodox therapies such as drugs or surgery? Or do these interfere with the action of prayer?

• Are some prayer strategies better than others? Is there a "best" way to pray?

• How about the skills of the people who pray? Does a spectrum of talent exist? Can prayer ability be acquired or is it innate?

• What conditions facilitate the effects of prayer, and which retard them?

• Is the effect of prayer always positive, or can it hurt as well as help?

These are the questions a scientist would be interested in asking, and that we shall pursue in this book.

"But however badly needed a good book on prayer is, I shall never try to write it," C. S. Lewis once said. "[In] a book one would inevitably seem to be attempting, not discussion, but instruction. And for me to offer the world instruction about prayer would be impudence."[9] I largely agree. How can one human being presume to know how another should approach the Absolute?

I therefore want the reader to know at the outset that this is not a "how to" book on prayer. These already exist in abundance. Rather this book is the result of my attempt to set aside everything I previously believed about prayer—to suspend, as much as possible, all judgments and assumptions, both positive and negative, about the subject—and simply to see what the record shows when focused through the lens of science and guided by thoughtful reason.

I am not an authority on prayer, nor do I pretend to be. If there is any justification for a physician addressing this subject, it is that both religious professionals and scientists currently appear to be poorly informed about the empirical evidence surrounding prayer. I am convinced that ignoring this body of knowledge leaves too much unsaid—particularly since so much of the evidence is positive. Neglecting this information results in an incomplete theology and a misshapen medicine, and it is bad science as well.

How can one remain silent on the place of spiritual issues, including prayer, in modern life? Skirting the spiritual has had a shattering effect on every dimension of contemporary existence. As England's great poet Kathleen Raine recently remarked, "Our society has lost the dimension of meanings and values—one could say the sacred—not only in the arts but in life itself."[10] Neglecting the sacred also bodes poorly, I am convinced, for the future. As novelist and philosopher André Malraux put it, "The twenty-first century will be religious or it will not be at all."[11]

Never did I believe that my search as a physician into the dynamics of healing would lead to an investigation of prayer—a subject whose enormity and majesty I acknowledge as our journey begins.

LARRY DOSSEY, M.D.
Santa Fe, New Mexico

PART 1

UNDERSTANDING

PRAYER AND HEALING

Chapter 1

Saints and Sinners, Health and Illness

> What is to give light must endure burning.
> —Viktor Frankl

One of the most puzzling illnesses in history took place some 2,500 years ago when the Buddha—the Awakened One—died from food poisoning, having been fed tainted meat in what proved to be his final meal. Not a very exalted way for a *Buddha* to go, I thought, on first discovering this account. Somehow I'd expected a more dignified cause of death than spoiled food. Later I found that this case was by no means unique, and that many great spiritual leaders have suffered ignominious ends marked by grotesque pain and suffering. Some of the historically recent examples include:

• Saint Bernadette, who in 1858 saw the vision of the Virgin at Lourdes, where thousands of healings are claimed to have occurred. Bernadette didn't receive such a healing when she needed one. Cause of death: variously called "bone cancer" or disseminated tuberculosis, at age thirty-five.

• Jiddu Krishnamurti, the famous spiritual teacher whose words have inspired millions around the world. Cause of death: cancer of the pancreas.

• Suzuki Roshi, who brought Zen Buddhism from Japan to the United States and established the San Francisco Zen Center. Cause of death: cancer of the liver.

• Sri Ramana Maharshi, the most beloved saint of modern India. Cause of death: cancer of the stomach.

This list could be multiplied at great length. History is clear: the health records of many of the most majestic, God-realized saints and mystics are far from ideal.

Often the sickly saints seem to accept illness as part of the natural order. The great Indian sage Sri Aurobindo, (1872–1950) one day took a wrong step, fell, and broke his knee. This perplexed the physician who attended him. "How is it that you, a mahatma, could not foresee and prevent this accident?" "I still have to carry this human body about me," Aurobindo replied, "and it is subject to ordinary human limitations and physical laws."[1]

The "explanations" offered for these events are numerous. Some say the saint or mystic wasn't *really* as spiritual as he or she seemed. Or that he or she was indeed enlightened but was living out his or her karma, "paying back" for transgressions and shortcomings of previous lives. Others maintain that the great teacher has inadvertently taken on the illness of his or her devotees, like an unconscious sponge. We also hear the argument that the wise one has consciously chosen the illness. Sometimes this is done as a teaching device, in order to demonstrate that the connection between the divine and the human can remain even in the midst of hideous illness. Or the saint or mystic intentionally takes on the illness as a final test, to "burn off" any remaining vestiges of ego or self-consciousness.[2]

These may or may not be valid reasons. Our task here is not to figure out in every case why God-realized people get sick and die, but simply to acknowledge that they obviously do—and to ask what this might imply when illness occurs in our own lives. Above all, these accounts should make us question seriously the prevalent assumptions that (a) being holy is a guarantee of good health, and that (b) bad health and illness always imply spiritual shortcomings.[3]

These assumptions are untrue not just for spiritual geniuses, but also for common folk like you and me. When Jesus encountered a man who was blind from birth, his disciples asked, "Master, who did sin, this man, or his parents, that he was born blind?" This question comes in a variety of "New Age" contexts today. Who is at fault? Why did I "choose" this illness? For what current or previous shortcomings am I suffering? Who's to blame? Jesus' answer is illuminating, and should be emblazoned in every New Age book dealing with consciousness and healing: "*Neither hath this man sinned, nor his parents:* but that the works of God should be made manifest in him" (John 9:1–3, King James Version [KJV], emphasis added). How could Jesus' message be clearer? This is a striking example of a profound physical problem in the total *absence* of spiritual imperfection. No one fell short, nobody was being punished for sin, nobody chose to be sick. Jesus implies also that there may be a higher purpose to the illness that we simply cannot grasp because we do not know the ways of the Absolute. This means that the meaning of a particular disease may be *cosmic*—that is, it may be opaque and hidden to us mortals, known only to the Divine. On balance, this case warns against equating spiritual and physical health, and cautions us against attributing shallow, superficial meaning to illness.

But the sickly saints and mystics are only one side of the coin. They are mirrored by what we could call the healthy reprobates—individuals who have no obvious spiritual inclinations whatever, but who never get sick. Almost everyone knows or has heard of such a person. They break all the rules of good health, smoke and drink with abandon, and live to be a hundred without ever falling ill.

Sickly saints and healthy sinners show us that there is no invariable, linear, one-to-one relationship between one's level of spiritual attainment and the degree of one's physical health. It is obvious that one can attain immense spiritual heights and still get *very* sick.

Many people who believe in an invariable relationship between physical health and spiritual attainment accept the concept of "the Divine within," the belief that an element or quality of the Supreme Being dwells inside every human. But even though the Divine may be present in everyone, it is obvious that human beings are imperfect reflectors, as it were, of the Divine Light. We fall short every day in a million ways. Just as we may contain an element of the Divine, our physical bodies may contain something of our spiritual essence, which they sometimes reflect as imperfectly as we reflect the Divine. When we fail to embody perfectly the Absolute, we do not say that God "sinned" or fell short;

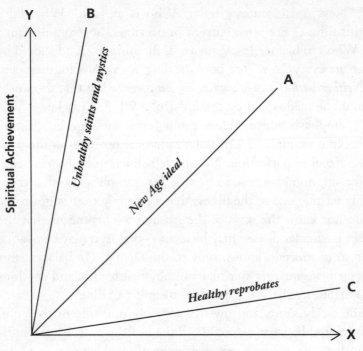

Figure 1

The level of spiritual achievement is plotted along the Y axis, and the degree of physical health is plotted along the X axis. The New Age ideal—the notion that spiritual achievement and physical health are always correlated—is illustrated by line A. This notion presupposes that for every gain in spirituality there is a corresponding gain in physical health, without exception—a one-to-one, straight-line, linear, invariant relationship. That this is not the case is illustrated by lines B and C. Line B shows that saints and mystics may be high spiritual achievers but may have poor physical health. Line C illustrates the opposite: people with little spiritual sensitivity—so-called spiritual reprobates—can enjoy extremely good physical health.

why then do we insist that a breakdown at the level of the body always implies that we erred? Physical bodies are obstreperous, stubborn entities that are given to some very bad habits, such as their susceptibility to genetic diseases, proneness to infection, and so on. Bodies have "minds of their own," which do not always accurately represent our psychological and spiritual understanding. Our bodies can act up, break down, and get sick without ever consulting us. Failure to recognize the relative intractability of the flesh is one of the excesses of today's consciousness-and-health movement, and is the potential cause of immense guilt when things go wrong.

A quick look at nature might help counter this problem. Plants, animals, birds, and fishes get sick, just as we do. In many instances they develop illnesses quite similar to our own, including cancer, arthritis, and bacterial and viral infections. They run headlong into accidents and trauma, and they too have the problems of old age and senility. Yet when animals or plants get sick, we take a different attitude toward them. We do not judge or blame them. We do not say that a tree is less a tree because it develops cancer or is infested with borers. It is not a dog's "fault" that it develops hip dysplasia, and a cat is not innately defective because it comes down with feline leukemia. In nature the occurrence of disease is considered a part of the natural order, not a sign of ethical, moral, or spiritual weakness.

We honor all living things in the midst of their sickness except ourselves. Most New Agers would never think of blaming their favorite rosebush when it becomes infected with aphids, but are quick to turn an accusing spotlight on themselves when they come down with strep throat. We are a part of nature no less than other creatures. The kindness, forgiveness, and gentleness we extend to them when they develop disease could well be extended to ourselves.

This is not to deny a general correlation between our physical and spiritual states. But we should not equate "general" with "invariable." In any given case, we simply may not know why serious illness develops.

STANDING IN THE MYSTERY

Our understanding of the relationship between spirituality and healing is vastly incomplete. We should admit the obvious:

There is great mystery here. By "mystery" I do not mean temporary ignorance that will later be swept away by additional information, or questions that will someday be resolved by future research. I mean mystery
in the strongest possible sense—something unknowable, something essentially beyond human understanding. The fact that saints sometimes
suffer and sinners don't is but one expression of this mystery; we shall
see many others unfolding throughout this book—such as the paradoxical power of praying for nothing instead of for something specific; the
power of the unconscious instead of the conscious mind in bringing
about healing; the fact that the effects of prayer, although demonstrable
in the laboratory, are agonizingly unpredictable outside it; and many
others.

Mystery irritates; it demands solutions. Perhaps this is because we
are so intolerant of ambiguity, generally preferring things in black or
white without shades of gray. When faced with mystery, we often engage in desperate attempts to solve it. The desperation is apparent, as
we've already seen, in the effort to explain away the occurrence of severe illness in spiritually enlightened individuals—*anything* to preserve
our preferred theory that good people don't get sick.

If we are ever to understand the role of prayer in healing, and the
relationship between spirituality and health, we shall have to grow
more tolerant of ambiguity and mystery. We shall have to be willing to
stand in the unknown.

THE PATHLESS PATH

There is no answer.
There never has been an answer.
There never will be an answer.
That's the answer.

—Gertrude Stein

The Grail legend is perhaps the quintessential Western
hero myth. As recounted by mythologist Joseph Campbell,[4] King
Arthur and his knights were gathered together at a banquet. The king
would not let the festivities begin until an adventure had occurred,
which was not long in coming. Suddenly, magically, the Holy Grail ap-

peared before all present. But it was draped and could not fully be seen, and then it disappeared. Gawain, Arthur's nephew, proposed that the knights go on a quest to find the Grail and view it fully, to which they all agreed. They recognized, however, that it would be a disgrace for them to embark on the search in a group. The decision was therefore made that each knight would pursue his quest alone, entering the forest at the place he alone had chosen, which to him seemed darkest, and where there was no path or guide.[5]

Campbell considered the Grail legend one of the most fundamental and powerful of Western myths, describing something deeply important about the workings of the Western mind. If he is correct, we Westerners do have the collective wisdom and ability to transcend all advice and rules in our search for matters of ultimate importance—no light, no path, no guide.

During illness we almost always want to enter the forest of therapy at a place chosen by someone else—a physician or health guru—where it is brightest, where there is a well-trodden path, and where guides and rules already exist. We want to eliminate ambiguity and uncertainty; we want only to know what works. We talk incessantly about practicalities, results, the "bottom line." In short we want a formula, one that tells us what to do.

The impulse to *do* when sick is understandable—to take the antibiotic with a cold's first sniffles, to rush to surgery, and so on—and a certain amount of doing is always valuable and can even be lifesaving. But doing must also be supplemented by *being*—looking inward, examining, focusing, wondering, asking. Being and doing are not incompatible; they can and should coexist. And for some people the most effective way to reverse illness is sometimes to focus primarily on being, following the Formula of No Formula, the Formula of Being Genuinely Who You Are, in which doing recedes into the background. Sometimes action will eventually emerge from this nonformula; if it does it will be authentic and natural and should be honored. The point is that action need not always be shoved reflexively and forcefully into the foreground as an automatic first-and-only choice when sick.

In 1987 I experienced the worst pain I've ever known. Like my father and twin brother before me, I had developed a herniated disc in the lumbar area. The pain was so intense I could neither walk nor stand. A lumbar myelogram and computerized tomography (CT) scan showed that the pain was caused by a bulging disc trapping a nerve leading into the left lower extremity. I consulted an expert neurologist and a skilled neurosurgeon. Their advice: Get off your feet and go to bed. If things aren't better in a month, have surgery to remove the disc. Things got worse. Even in bed the slightest movement would trigger waves of pain that were almost unbearable.

Through the years I had become increasingly visible in my community as a spokesman for the role of consciousness in health. I had written books on the subject that were widely read. As a consequence I knew most of the practitioners of alternative forms of health care in my area. When they heard of my difficulty, they came to my aid by the dozens. I quickly found myself surrounded by wonderful friends, all of whom wanted to use their special techniques to help me recover. My wife had to resort to a formal scheduling procedure to manage the constant stream of healers. Acupuncturists, psychic healers, prayer therapists, homeopaths, "body workers" of various sorts, nutritionists, hands-on healers, craniosacral therapists, osteopaths, and chiropractors—all came to my assistance. They employed a wide variety of techniques and tools: needles, magnets, crystals, pyramids, copper electrodes, and colored lights. I delighted in all these therapies. Even though some seemed zany, I didn't care. I was grateful for the love, compassion, and attention my friends freely gave me.

Eventually, however, my feelings changed. I began to experience an intense craving for solitude. I needed time to be alone and think about what was happening. To my surprise I began to resent the bright, sunny, positive assurances that I'd be well in no time; that everything would have a happy ending; that each particular therapy was the key to my healing.

One day my dear friend Jeanne Achterberg called. I had not seen her in months. Dr. Achterberg is a first-rate bioscientist in the field of psychophysiology; with her husband, Dr. G. Frank Lawlis, she had done pioneer work in how mental imagery affects the body. "Getting tired of all the 'therapy'?" Jeanne asked. "I went through this years ago," she continued. "Eventually I felt like a big jungle cat who is injured. I wanted to hide in a dark cave deep in the jungle, completely hidden, and simply lick my wounds. I wanted to remain there, letting things be, until my situation resolved itself—one way or the other." Jeanne was reading my mind. She helped me acknowledge my increasing resistance to the ministrations of my friends. I soon found myself withdrawing from their support. I was in my own cave, licking my wounds.

Many of my friends did not appreciate my need to withdraw. Some implied that I was not "facilitating" my own cure; that I was courting illness by not fighting back; that I was unconsciously choosing to be sick. As the pain and disability grew steadily worse, I decided to have surgery. This was the final straw for a few of these friends, who viewed my choice as a sellout to "modern medicine." They felt I should have persisted with the less invasive, mind-oriented approaches. I only knew that I was tired of the pain, that I'd given alternative methods a good try, and that it was time to move on.

The period of withdrawal and solitude was highly illuminating for me. I kept an extensive journal, and my wife rigged a bedside table that enabled me to use my word processor while flat in bed. The weeks of pain proved ironically to be one of the most fertile writing periods of my life. I managed to finish a lengthy book project, as new ideas flowed from some invisible source. I began to realize that this immensely trying experience had a hidden dimension that was not all bad. I wondered if my book would have remained unfinished had I continued to receive alternative treatments. Would the fresh insights have been aborted? Would my understanding of the meaning of my illness have been blocked?

I realized there were benefits to feeling bad—but I found it almost impossible to communicate this idea to others. It was invariably interpreted as a morbid focusing on pain, relishing illness, courting disease; I was languishing in my problems. I was certain that more was involved, something that Germany's great poet Rainer Maria Rilke struggled to describe:

> So you must not be frightened . . . if a sadness rises up before you larger than any you have ever seen; if a restiveness, like light and cloud-shadows, passes over your hands and over all you do. You must think that . . . life has not forgotten you, that it holds you in its hand; it will not let you fall. Why do you want to shut out of your life any agitation, any pain, any melancholy, since you really

do not know what these states are working upon you? Why do you want to persecute yourself with the question whence all this may be coming and whither it is bound? . . . just remember that sickness is the means by which an organism frees itself of foreign matter; so one must just help it to be sick, to have its whole sickness and break out with it, for that is its progress. . . . you must be patient as a sick man. . . . there are in every illness many days when the doctor can do nothing but wait. And this it is that you, insofar as you are your own doctor, must now above all do.[6]

Rilke knew there were inner meanings and messages to illness. If illness were never experienced, or if it were banished at its earliest appearance by medication or surgery—or if it were immediately "prayed away"—this wisdom might never be gained.

Even the *willingness* to experience pain, the *acceptance* of unpleasantness, can transform them into something else. An example comes from author Natalie Goldberg, who gives writing workshops around the country. When she finished her book *Writing Down the Bones* in Santa Fe in 1984, she felt the need to visit her great Buddhist teacher Katagiri Roshi in Minneapolis, with whom she had previously studied for six years. She showed him the book and said, "Roshi, I need a teacher again. The people in Santa Fe are crazy. They drift from one thing to another."

"Don't be so greedy," he replied, shaking his head. "Writing is taking you very deep. Continue to write."

"But Roshi, it is so lonely."

"Is there anything wrong with loneliness?" he asked, lifting his eyebrows.

"No, I guess not."

The conversation went to other things. Suddenly she interrupted him. "But Roshi, you have sentenced me to such loneliness. Writing is very lonely," she stressed again.

"Anything you do deeply is very lonely," he replied.

"Are you lonely?" she asked him.

"Of course," he answered. "But I do not let it toss me away. It is just loneliness."[7]

The terminal cancer of Ramana Maharshi perplexed many of his followers who had left everything to go to India to study at his ashram. Many questioned their decision, for surely such an enlightened master should not be dying from such a common disease. Maharshi's pain was immense; he would scream out at night, disturbing the entire community. When someone would accidentally bump into him, a look of great misery would flash across his face. He made no comment about these moments, however, until someone, thinking he was using yogic control, said to him, "Perhaps you don't feel the pain?" "There is pain," Maharshi responded, "but there is no suffering." His followers received a lesson in how one can stand in the illness and transform pain and agony, while not avoiding or eradicating it.[8]

The idea that bliss and happiness are our "birthright," that when we recognize our own "inner divinity" we shall be perpetually happy, is very popular today for obvious reasons. For proof adherents point to the few mortals who claim to have attained this state. But many spiritual masters believe that God is not "pure bliss," "pure love," or pure anything. They maintain that God is unknowable. God is also undefinable, because attaching any characteristic to the Infinite excludes its opposite, immediately violating the wholeness and completeness of the Absolute, outside of which nothing can exist. Among the spiritual geniuses who took the position that God is not just "the good things," such as bliss, happiness, pleasure, and health, was the thirteenth-century German mystic Meister Eckhart, who wrote,

> Some people want to recognize God only in some pleasant enlightenment—and then they get pleasure and enlightenment but not God.[9]

PRAYER AND PRAYERFULNESS

During illness the quiet way of being we've been examining flows from one's true center. It is focused, authentic, genuine, and accepting of any outcome. It is not self-conscious and contains no pity for the "I" who is sick. It is not contaminated by fear of death, and contains no blame or guilt. It does not exclude any therapeutic approach, and may involve using drugs or surgery as naturally as contemplation, meditation, or prayer. It is unconcerned with tragic outcomes, even death, for it rests in the understanding that one's higher Self is immortal and eternal, and cannot die.

We should not equate these ways of being with doing nothing. Beneath the tranquility, equanimity, and acceptance lies a kind of action that bears little resemblance to the showy activity to which we are accustomed. This quiet, inner-directed action is acknowledged in many spiritual traditions as the highest form of activity in which humans can engage, and is almost identical with some forms of prayer.

Prayer, as we shall see, takes many forms. Many people follow the formalities of the great religions and pray explicitly for specific events to occur. Some people pray to a personal God or Goddess, the Almighty, or Supreme Being, others to an impersonal Universe or the Absolute. Others do not pray in any conventional sense, but live with a deeply interiorized sense of the sacred. Theirs could be called a spirit of prayerfulness, a sense of simply being attuned or aligned with "something higher."

Prayer tends to follow instructions laid down by the great religious traditions; prayerfulness does not. It is a feeling of unity with the All, rather than with specific leaders, traditions, or holy books. Intercessory prayer has a tendency to ask for definite outcomes, to structure the future, to "tell God what to do," such as taking the cancer away. Prayerfulness, on the other hand, is accepting without being passive, is grateful without giving up. It is more willing to stand in the mystery, to tolerate ambiguity and the unknown. It honors the rightness of whatever happens, even cancer.

Many action-oriented people equate prayerfulness with inactivity, giving in, and giving up. (Later we'll see that this attitude seems to originate in rather fixed, innate personality tendencies and has little to do with spirituality.) They may even accuse inner-directed, prayerful people of "doing nothing" in the face of illness and crisis. Most contemplative people have borne the brunt of this criticism at some time in their lives. It can be harshest when they are sick. When faced with someone else's heart disease, cancer, or some other serious medical problem, action-oriented friends seem to come out of the woodwork with action-packed advice. They seem concerned only about what the sick person should do, not about how he or she should be.

This is nothing new. There seems always to have been an unbridgeable gap separating outer-directed actives and inner-directed contemplatives. A description of this perennial difference in perspective is given in *The Cloud of Unknowing*, an influential, anonymously written religious document that emerged in fourteenth-century England:

> Just as when Martha complained of Mary her sister, so to this day do actives complain of contemplatives. Wherever you find anyone . . . who feels moved through God's grace and guidance to forsake all outward activity and set about living the contemplative life . . . just as soon will you find his brothers, sisters, best friends, and sundry others, who know nothing of his inward urge, or the contemplative life itself, rise up with great complaint, and sharply reprove him, and tell him he is wasting his time. And they will recount all sorts of tales, some false and some true, describing how men and women who have given themselves up to such a life in the past have fallen. There is never a tale of those who make good.[10]

Yet activity and the struggle to be healed are also natural. Many wild creatures know the right plants or herbs to eat when they are sick. Prayerfully honoring one's place in the natural order does not necessarily mean accepting disease passively without a fight. But sometimes the struggle leads to insights that transcend the presence or absence of specific illnesses, and generates an understanding that could be called "higher health"—the certain knowledge that health and illness can paradoxically coexist.[11]

If we allow ourselves to enter the quiet, still place of prayerfulness, we can understand the co-relationship of health and illness in the natural order; we can sense how John Updike could say, with wide-eyed astonishment and gratitude, "We do survive every moment, after all, except the last one."[12]

In *The Spirituality of Imperfection*, historian Ernest Kurtz and writer Katherine Ketcham relate an Islamic story that illustrates the intense degree of gratitude that is possible even in the midst of illness:

> Sa'ad son of Wakas was a companion of the Prophet. In his last years he became blind and settled in Mecca, where he was always

surrounded by people seeking his blessing. He did not bless everyone, but those whom he did always found the way smoothed for
them.

Abdallah Ibn-Sa'ad reports:

"I went to see him, and he was good to me and gave me his blessing. As I was only a curious child, I asked him: 'Your prayers for
others always seem to be answered. Why, then, do you not pray
for your blindness to be removed?'

"The ancient replied: 'Submission to the Will of God is far
better than the personal pleasure of being able to see.'"[13]

After reading my book *Beyond Illness*, which explores the paradox
of the coexistence of health and illness, a woman wrote:

When I was a small child, my sister and I used to play a game we
invented called Perfect Leaf. We would go into the backyard and
search diligently for a leaf on any tree or shrub that was perfect.
The first person to find one was the winner. This may sound un-
believable, but the game could go on for hours, particularly in late
summer and fall. By then almost all the leaves were imperfect—
chewed by insects, shriveled on the edges, marred in endless ways.

Perfect Leaf was more than a game. It taught us a lesson we
didn't know we were learning at the time—that beauty and ugli-
ness, perfection and imperfection, can coexist—not only in the
same leaf, but probably in ourselves as well.[14]

This lesson seems all but forgotten today. For example, one of the
most common New Age exercises for promoting a state of perfect health
is to visualize "pure white light" washing over one's body. Most people
who do this do not realize that both "white light" and "perfect health"
are illusions. Light is white only because it contains many different col-
ors and hues—the entire visible spectrum—not because it is "pure."
Health, like light, is also a mixture, because human experience is made
possible only through contrasts. "Experience" requires "difference."
This means that health, like light, cannot be pure; it must contain an el-

ement of illness to be experienced at all. Philosopher Alan Watts expressed the point trenchantly. "Because human consciousness must involve both pleasure and pain," he wrote, "to strive for pleasure to the exclusion of pain is, in effect, to strive for loss of consciousness."[15]

To totally purify health through prayer, meditation, or anything else is to destroy it. "Perfect health" is a contradiction in terms.

THE POWER OF PRAYERFULNESS

One night, following a lecture I gave on health and healing, a woman came forward to speak to me. Clearly shy, she had held back until the auditorium was almost empty. Looking around to make sure no one else was listening, she said almost in a whisper that thirty years ago she had been diagnosed with metastatic cancer. What did she do to get rid of it? *Nothing*, she revealed. She went on to say that nobody wanted to hear her story; that people like her never get interviewed on "Oprah" or "Donahue," which seem interested only in those dramatic cases where people do heroic, colorful things.

She is right. Almost all the books that have emerged in recent years on the subject describe how to "beat" cancer with aggressive actions of an astonishing variety. Discussing the role of prayerfulness and "doing nothing" is about as enticing as announcing on the ten o'clock news that all the planes landed safely today at LaGuardia or O'Hare. This is unfortunate, because there is increasing evidence that prayerfulness can save lives.

Prayerfulness—not the world-manipulating, disease-bashing forms of prayer to which most Westerners resort when sick—permeates many cases of profound illness that improve spontaneously. Prayerfulness allows us to reach a plane of experience where illness can be experienced as a natural part of life, and where its acceptance transcends passivity. If the disease disappears, we are grateful; if it remains, that too is reason for gratitude.

The "attitude of gratitude" during illness is captured in the following curious story in which the disease went away—part of the time.

At the turn of the twentieth century there was a religious group in Mysore, India, headed by a famous holy man. He was afflicted with chills from malaria, a common affliction in those days. His bodily shaking was so severe it would interfere with his prayers.

The swami used to take his morning bath in the temple pond. Then, wearing his wet two-piece garment he would go to the sanctum sanctorum to offer prayers. When the chills got particularly bad he would remove the wet cloth covering his upper body and toss it in a corner. The wet garment would continue to shiver and shake while the swami would be free of chills and able to offer his prayers. Once his prayers were completed he would pick up the cloth from the corner and again wrap it around himself, which would bring the shivers back to him.

When asked why he did not leave off the cloth permanently, thereby never having to have chills again, he replied that it was a sufficient blessing that for short periods he could get away from his physical symptoms so he could perform his ritual worship.[16]

SPONTANEOUS REGRESSION OF CANCER

My present purpose is not to vaunt a new remedy but to state a fact—that cancer, even when advanced in degree and of long duration, may get better, and does sometimes get well. *There is cure of cancer,* apart from operative removal. . . . These cases . . . are the sun of our hope.[17]

—Sir Alfred Pearce Gould (1910)

The patron saint for spontaneous regression of cancers is St. Peregrine. While a young priest, he was scheduled for amputation of his leg because of a cancer. The night before surgery, he prayed fervently and dreamed he was cured. On awakening his dream had become reality. He lived to be eighty, dying in 1345 without any further evidence of cancer. During his long life he dedicated himself to serving those afflicted with such problems, and was canonized St. Peregrine in 1726. Dr. William Boyd, professor emeritus of pathology at the University of Toronto and an authority on the spontaneous regression of cancer, has suggested that tumors that disappear spontaneously be called "St. Peregrine tumors."[18]

How often does cancer spontaneously regress, leaving the person healthy? Opinions vary. Researchers T. C. Everson and W. H. Cole collected 176 case reports from various countries around the world on spontaneous regression of cancer (SRC), and concluded that SRC occurs in one out of 100,000 cases of cancer.[19] Other authorities believe the incidence may be higher, perhaps one in 80,000 cases.

If these statistics are true, SRC is uncommon, to say the least. Thus if SRC is indeed "the sun of our hope," it is a sun that does not shine very brightly.

In analyzing their 176 cases of SRC, Everson and Cole found that almost *any* therapy seems to work *some* of the time. Regression of cancer followed such diverse measures as intercessory prayer, conversion to Christian Science, mud packs, vitamin therapy, and force-feeding. SRC has even been reported following electroshock treatments to the brain, and following coma induced by the administration of insulin. These researchers concluded that, since almost any treatment seemed to work occasionally but not consistently, all these measures were equally worthless and that SRC is purely a random event entirely beyond the control of an individual patient. According to this point of view, the disappearance of St. Peregrine's cancer had nothing to do with prayer; it would have happened anyway for reasons that are essentially obscure and unpredictable. The saint was simply one of the lucky ones. And in any case, these events are too rare to hold out as hope to people suffering from cancer, especially since they cannot control them.

This forlorn point of view, although currently popular, is a historical oddity. Prior to our century, physicians and patients alike commonly believed that the mind was a major factor in the development and course of cancer. Only in recent times has this opinion changed.[20] Is there anything in current medical research that might justify a return to the belief in the "powers of the mind"? The question of the role of the psyche in cancer is complex, and it isn't our purpose to review it here. Our subject is prayer and its possible role in healing. I therefore want to cite several cases that strongly suggest that it can be an important factor in the course of cancer.

In 1975 professor and physician Yujiro Ikemi and his colleagues at Kyushu University's School of Medicine in Fukuoka, Japan, reported five cases of SRC. Although these cases come from Japan, that does not make them exotic or special; similar cases can be found in all cultures. I have chosen them for a specific reason. Looking at cases outside our own society can illuminate key features in the regression process that we ordinarily don't notice—such as the role played by prayerfulness.

Ikemi and his co-workers selected these cases prospectively and unselectively according to strict criteria. This means the researchers did not "skim off the top," picking only cases that conformed to their expectations and preconceived ideas. The reports are scientifically precise and include biopsy confirmation of all the cancers in question. On balance these remarkable cases seem to contradict the idea that SRC is accidental, random, and beyond the effects of a patient's thoughts, attitudes, and feelings. They strongly suggest that there is a profound effect of prayerfulness and an indwelling spiritual sense on the cancer process.[21]

In order to be considered an example of spontaneous regression, a case had to meet strict criteria generally accepted by cancer researchers. These criteria do not equate SRC with "cure," which implies the total disappearance of the cancer. The cancer may remain; it simply does not take a toll on the patient's health. He or she remains alive and well, with cancer along for the ride.

Ikemi's first case involved Y. H., a male church worker who was born on a farm in Japan in 1886. (Ikemi's remaining four cases of spontaneous regression are described in Appendix 2.) At age eighteen he became a member of the Shinto religious sect, and at age twenty-one he was appointed a teacher in his church. Thereafter he was promoted to district leader of the organization and devoted his future life to church work.

The Shinto religion experienced a great crisis during World War II. During this time Y. H.'s responsibilities were increased immensely. In addition to his church work, he was asked to take over important business involving the administration of his town. A self-punitive and taciturn person by nature, he found it very difficult to cope with all these responsibilities.

In March 1950, when he was sixty-four years old, Y. H. noticed the sudden appearance of nasal obstruction and bleeding while at work. He was referred to specialists at the medical school at Kyushu University, where his evaluation resulted in a biopsy and the diagnosis of a cancer of the right maxilla, or upper jaw. The tumor was resected in April.

His problems were not over. In January of the following year, he developed hoarseness and a dry feeling in his throat. He thought he had caught a cold, but eventually a new cancer was discovered on the left vocal cord, again confirmed by biopsy.

The medical school specialists recommended radical surgery— the removal of his larynx, including the vocal cords—but Y. H. declined. He stated that he preferred continuing to be a preacher for as long as he could speak to losing his voice from the surgery. "This is God's will and I have no complaint about it," he felt. "Whatever should happen will just happen."

Ten days after he received his "sentence of cancer," he went to see the president of his religious organization. "Remember that you are an invaluable asset for our church," the leader told him. This left Y. H. extremely happy; he shed tears of joy all the way home. Beginning with this experience, his hoarseness improved. Four months later he began to give short speeches at his church again. Two months later he could speak for up to thirty minutes and his voice was quite clear.

Y. H. lived for the next thirteen years without any form of medical treatment or surgery. Repeated evaluation revealed no evidence of the laryngeal tumor. He died at age seventy-eight from an unrelated cause— trauma to his back, which led to his general deterioration.

This case has several notable features. Following his diagnosis Y. H. showed no tendency to lapse into depression, despair, lack of motivation, and fear of death, which is typical of many patients. He did not engage in specific prayers in which he pleaded or bargained with God to "change the diagnosis" and grant him a cure. He did not "fight" cancer in any ordinary sense of the word, as doctors and others often recommend today. His attitude was rather one of renewed commitment and gratitude to God, combined with the belief that God's will was being done, no matter what happened.

Y. H.'s case demonstrates a paradoxical theme that runs through all the examples reported by Ikemi: *Often a prayerful, prayer-like attitude of devotion and acceptance—not robust, aggressive prayer for specific outcomes, including eradication of the cancer—precedes the cure.*

Ikemi's work seems to indicate that cancers sometimes regress spontaneously, not when some specific formula is followed, but when all formulas are abandoned. "Formula" is derived from the Latin *forma*, or form. These patients were not following some formula designed to banish cancer—not taking on someone else's form, not adopting behaviors they'd heard about or observed to work in the cancer experiences of others. They were simply and authentically being themselves, honoring the experiences that emerged from their own psychic depths.

Neither did they follow some "spiritual formula" *in order to* rid themselves of cancer. On becoming ill many people adopt a spiritual way of being with a hidden agenda: to rid themselves of disease. The Japanese cases show, however, that spirituality is not a commodity to be used during illness, like a drug. To use spirituality for a specific purpose would be a contradiction in terms, an exercise in hypocrisy. Get-well formulas that advocate spiritual practices are by definition inauthentic because they require that one take on spirituality from the outside, instead of allowing it to emerge from the center of one's being.

The Japanese cases suggest therefore that the key in regression may lie in simply being true to oneself. In order to do this genuinely, one must go beyond all formulas, all paths, all programs, and give up all ulterior wishes—including, perhaps, the hope that the cancer disappears.

This is admittedly a very difficult and unpopular task. People who are ill don't want to hear advice of this sort. They want specific, nononsense steps to take—the formula—that will banish the disease. Perhaps the difficulty and unpopularity of these measures is a reason why spontaneous regression of cancer is not more common.

BEATING ILLNESS: IS THERE A FORMULA?

This cannot be expressed, cannot be narrowed into words, cannot be subjected to laws; every man is completely free and has his own special liberation. . . . No form of instruction exists, no Savior exists to open up the road. No road exists to be opened.

—Nikos Kazantzakis, *The Saviors of God*[22]

> There is a type of person in whose mind God is always
> mixed up with vitamins.
>
> —Manly P. Hall[23]

What if a person with cancer tried intentionally to du-
plicate the key features in the Japanese cases above? What if he or she
deliberately adopted an attitude of prayerfulness, gratitude, and acceptance; eliminated anxiety and depression; experienced an existential
shift following diagnosis; and patched up his or her interpersonal relationships? Would the cancer go away? Can we derive a formula from
cases of spontaneous regression of cancer that everyone could employ
successfully?

Many Western-trained physicians believe there must be some
common technique that all cancer patients could use to rid themselves
of cancer—if only we could discover it. Physician and writer Lewis
Thomas, for instance, has said,

> The rare but spectacular phenomenon of spontaneous remission
> of cancer patients persists in the annals of medicine, . . . a fascinat-
> ing mystery, but at the same time a solid basis for hope in the fu-
> ture: if several hundred patients have succeeded in doing this sort
> of thing, eliminating vast numbers of malignant cells on their
> own, the possibility that medicine can learn to accomplish the
> same thing at will is surely within reach of imagining.[24]

California physician and author Rachel Naomi Remen, whose
work with extremely ill and dying patients is widely known, believes
that such a formula does not currently exist. She states,

> I asked fifteen or twenty clinical colleagues if they could identify
> positive emotions in their patients—that is to say, emotions that
> they felt were directly associated with survival. There was no
> question that all these physicians and psychologists liked certain
> emotions better than others, but the correlation between survival
> and emotional attitude was not clear to any of them, including the
> oncologists. All had worked with loving, cheerful people who

died, grieving people who lived, angry people who never became ill, and humorous people who were unable to heal themselves. And yet all had the clinical hunch that emotions indeed affect healing. So we have a mystery. Perhaps we need more sensitive tools for studying emotional and psychological states. The sensitivity of our emotional assessment needs to equal the sophistication of our immunological knowledge, and we are not there yet.[25]

Our age is besotted with self-help formulas of a mind-boggling variety. The tabloids and talk shows tout the plan-of-the-week for weight loss, heightened sexual prowess, or elimination of cancer. The spell woven by all this blather is hypnotic. The tendency is always to accord wisdom to something or someone outside ourselves. The idea that we could bypass all the self-declared experts and consultants and focus on our internal healing strengths simply does not occur to most people. Even more rare is the insight that even if the cancer doesn't disappear, that too can be acceptable and "right."

This is in stark contrast to the advice delivered by many New Age health "authorities" who speak and write endlessly of the marvelous results one can expect if certain measures are aggressively undertaken to transform one's personality, relationships, goals, thought habits, philosophy, and overall orientation to life. This advice invariably implies that the cancer (or any other illness) has arisen because of imperfections in the patient's life. If he or she can somehow summon the courage and honesty to set the defects right, the miracle can take place. Invariably love, forgiveness, and openness are emphasized as crucial elements in this radical psychological and physical transformation. Some health gurus advise a kaleidoscopic array of other measures—diet, exercise, meditation, vitamins, herbs, body work, laughter, thinking positive thoughts—the list is virtually endless.

This approach is what Jungian psychologist James Hillman calls the "rainmaker fantasy"—the shamanic idea that once the rainmaker puts himself in order, the rain falls. Translated into New Age health thinking, "If I really straighten myself out, the disease will disappear."[26]

One reason this Promethean formula endures is because it cannot be proved wrong so long as one looks only at the experience of individual patients. If the cure does not occur, this is evidence not that the formula was wrong, but that the person did not try hard enough or did not really "want" to be cured. The failure of cure is explained thus not as a defect in the advice, but in the person following it.[27] Some people who follow these methods do experience cure; indeed anything appears to work some of the time. But when subjected to systematic scrutiny, these methods frequently do not hold up. In one controlled study, "exceptional" cancer patients who followed a rigorous formula of self-transformation did no better than "control" cancer patients treated conventionally—a side of the coin that is seldom admitted by self-help advocates.[28]

So far no one has been able to demonstrate that cancer or any other disease will predictably disappear by using prayer, meditation, or any psychological or spiritual method whatever. Michael Lerner, Ph.D., is president and founder of the Commonweal Cancer Help Program in California, which is devoted to service and research in health and human ecology. For a decade Lerner has researched alternative treatments for cancer and is perhaps the leading authority in the United States in this area. (He was special consultant to the U. S. Office of Technology Assessment in preparing its major report on Unconventional Cancer Treatments.) Following his decade-long investigation, Lerner has concluded that although there is plenty of anecdotal evidence that many such therapies improve the quality of life, he has not found any cure for cancer among the many unconventional methods he examined, and little scientific evidence that such methods extend life beyond what could be achieved with conventional treatments.[29]

Countless numbers of people who pray for diseases to go away would be utterly baffled and stunned should this actually happen. As Susan Ertz put it, "Millions long for immortality who do not know what to do with themselves on a rainy Sunday afternoon."[30] What on earth happened? Where did the cure come from? Why did it occur? What is the purpose of my healing? What am I to do with my life now that the disease has gone?

Even if prayer or attempts at self-transformation fail in the course of illness, there is still a sense in which a cure can always occur. By "cure" I do not mean the *physical* disappearance of cancer, heart disease, high blood pressure, or stroke, but something more marvelous—the realization that *physical illness, no matter how painful or grotesque, is at some level of secondary importance in the total scheme of our existence.* This is the awareness that one's authentic, higher self is completely impervious to the ravages of any physical ailment whatever. The disease may regress or totally disappear when this awareness dawns, for reasons we may not understand. When this happens it comes as a gift, a blessing, a grace—but again, this is of secondary importance. The real cure is the realization that at the most essential level, we are all "untouchables"—utterly beyond the ravages of disease and death.

We begin our journey into prayer and healing by acknowledging great mysteries that cannot be resolved by formulas and intellectualization. Honoring these great unknowns, we now take a closer look at how prayer manifests in our lives.

Chapter 2

The Reach of the Mind:
Setting the Stage for Prayer

What is your life, and whence, and where?
> —Nikos Kazantzakis, *The Odyssey:*
> *A Modern Sequel*

The psyche's attachment to the brain, i.e., its space-time limitation, is no longer as self-evident and incontrovertible as we have hitherto been led to believe.
. . . The fact that we are totally unable to imagine a form of existence without space and time by no means proves that such an existence is in itself impossible. . . . It is not only permissible to doubt the absolute validity of space-time perception; it is, in view of the available facts, even imperative to do so.

> —C. G. Jung, *Psychology and the Occult*

The intelligible, therefore, is not imprisoned within the body; it spreads in all the body's parts, it penetrates them, it goes through them, and could not be enclosed in any place.

> —Porphyry (ca. A.D. 233–305)

The idea that the human mind can affect the physical body has a long and honored history. We find in the two thousand-year-old *Hippocratic Writings* the observation that "there is a measure of

conscious thought throughout the body." The Persians took this attitude much further. They claimed that a person's mind can intervene
not just in his or her own body, but also in that of another individual
who might be quite far away. A thousand years ago, for example, the
legendary Persian physician Avicenna (A.D. 980–1037) stated, "The
imagination of a man can act not only on his own body but even others
and very distant bodies. It can fascinate and modify them; make them
ill, or restore them to health."[1]

These attitudes of the Greeks and Persians toward the relationship
between minds and bodies illustrate two very different types of healing.
For the Greeks the action of the mind on the body was a *local* event—
that is, it happened locally, in the here and now. Such a perspective implies that *my* mind is in *my* body, not in yours; and when it affects the
body, it is *mine* that is affected and nobody else's. In contrast the Persian
view of the mind-body relationship was *nonlocal:* my mind is not localized or confined to my body, but extends outside it. This suggests that it
is capable of affecting not only my own body, but other bodies that may
be very far way. The Persians were referring to a mind that is nonlocal in
space. But minds may be nonlocal in *time* as well as space, as we will see.

Modern medicine has made it quite unfashionable to think about
ideas like these. The possibility that a mind could be nonlocal, that it
might extend beyond an individual body, is now considered outrageous,
although in times past this was considered an appropriate concern for
physicians. We need to lift this embargo. *Every* physician, in the course
of practicing clinical medicine, becomes a collector of bizarre observations, cases that do not fit the norm, that he or she files away secretly
over the years. These observations can be as strange as anything
Avicenna proposed. They may be immensely troubling, and physicians
may be reluctant to discuss them. They may even try to dismiss them in
various ways, such as by using innocent-sounding terms to decontami-
nate them—calling them "the natural course of the illness" or "the statistical variation of the disease." When confronted by an unexpected
and unexplainable clinical variation, physicians will occasionally say,
"We see this"—as if these sorts of statements can magically annul the
strangeness of the happening. All these "explanations" are illusory.
They simply say, "What happens, happens."

CONCEPTS OF MEDICINE FROM 1860 TO THE PRESENT: ERAS I, II, AND III

In order to demonstrate that prayer-related healing fits into medical science, let's drop back to the nineteenth century, when medicine first began to become "scientific." This happened just around the time of the American Civil War, in the 1860s. Prior to that time, almost everything physicians did to help patients—leeching, bleeding, purging, for example—was either ineffective or actually harmful. (Ironically, many antiquated therapies seem to be making a comeback. The use of leeches, snake venom, bloodletting, and purging have been found to have a value in certain situations—but are used with greater insight and delicacy now than in the past.) But around this period the profession as a whole developed a strong case of "physics envy," wanting to embody the precision and predictability characteristic of that science. If we begin at that historical moment and come forward to the present, we can sort out three historical eras that embody fundamentally different approaches to the nature of health and illness and healing:

• Era I: the era of physicalistic medicine that dominated medicine from the 1860s to about 1950, and which is still influential

• Era II: the era of mind-body medicine that arose in the 1950s and which is still developing

• Era III: our era of nonlocal science and medicine, which is just being recognized.

Era I

Era I, which began in the last third of the nineteenth century, can be called the era of materialistic or physicalistic medicine. It encompasses the discovery and practice of therapies that largely dominate Western medicine today—drugs, surgery, radiation, and so on. Era I medicine is guided by the classical laws of matter and energy that Sir Isaac Newton described in the seventeenth century. According to these "laws," the entire universe, including the body, is a vast clockwork that functions according to deterministic, causal principles. If they are to be effective, all forms of therapy must embody these physicalistic

TABLE 2 **Medical Eras**

	ERA I
Space-Time Characteristic	Local
Synonym	Mechanical, material, or physical medicine
Description	Causal, deterministic, describable by classical concepts of space-time and matter-energy. Mind not a factor; "mind" a result of brain mechanisms.
Examples	Any form of therapy focusing solely on the effects of *things* on the body are Era I approaches—including techniques such as acupuncture and homeopathy, the use of herbs, etc. Almost all forms of "modern" medicine—drugs, surgery, irradiation, CPR, etc.—are included.

Table 2 shows the differences and similarities between Eras I, II, and III.

Era II	Era III
Local	Nonlocal
Mind-body medicine	Nonlocal or transpersonal medicine
Mind a major factor in healing *within* the single person. Mind has causal power; is thus not fully explainable by classical concepts in physics. Includes but goes beyond Era I.	Mind a factor in healing both *within* and *between* persons. Mind not completely localized to points in space (brains or bodies) or time (present moment or single lifetimes). Mind is unbounded and infinite in space and time—thus omnipresent, eternal, and ultimately unitary or one. Healing at a distance is possible. Not describable by classical concepts of space-time or matter-energy.
Any therapy emphasizing the effects of consciousness solely within the individual body is an Era II approach. Psychoneuroimmunology, counseling, hypnosis, biofeedback, relaxation therapies, and most types of imagery-based "alternative" therapies are included.	Any therapy in which effects of consciousness bridge between different persons is an Era III approach. All forms of distant healing, intercessory prayer, some types of shamanic healing, diagnosis at a distance, telesomatic events, and probably noncontact therapeutic touch are included.

assumptions. This means that in Era I the effects of mind and consciousness were considered of secondary importance, if of any importance at all.

Let there be no mistake: Era I medicine was enormously important in the history of healing. Its accomplishments are too numerous to name and they speak for themselves. These achievements are *so* significant that most people believe that the entire future of medicine lies in Era I approaches.

Era II

Sometime in the mid-twentieth century, in the years following World War II, another unique period in the history of Western medicine began to take shape—Era II, or "mind-body" medicine. Although mind-body approaches had existed since antiquity, at long last they began to be studied scientifically. As this field developed, it became possible to show that perceptions, emotions, attitudes, thoughts, and perceived meanings profoundly affect the body, sometimes dramatically.

This evidence is too vast to be reviewed here; yet a great many skeptics continue to claim that this body of research does not exist, that there is no evidence that the mind can affect the body in clinically relevant ways. There is, I feel, a quick cure for skeptics who do not believe in the legitimacy of Era II. They might visit a biofeedback laboratory, where it can be demonstrated in only a few moments that mind *can* move matter. It is possible to make meters move dramatically merely by willing, and to trigger bells and whistles on sophisticated electronic gadgetry *merely by taking thought*, by changing one's mental images and feeling states. Moreover these feats can be duplicated *on command*. It has also been shown conclusively that these mind-related changes are correlated with healthful changes in the body. On balance this evidence demonstrates that thoughts deserve, as genuinely as any drug or surgical procedure, to be called "therapeutic."[2]

Era II, or mind-body approaches to therapy, need not conflict with the physically based therapies of Era I. They can and often do complement one another, leading to entirely new disciplines such as the still-developing field of psychoneuroimmunology.

Eras I and II have much in common. For instance, they are both entirely *local* in emphasis—that is, both consider the mind to be localized to points in space (the brain and body) and time (the present moment). Consistent with the local view, Era II emphasizes the mind of the *single, individual* person operating on her or his own *individual* body, all within a classical, local, space-time framework.

Many enthusiasts of Era II believe that mind-body approaches are the ultimate form of therapy, and that healing can go no higher. But as important an advance as Era II medicine has been, we now can see that, like Era I medicine, it is also limited and incomplete, because there simply are too many healing events for which it cannot account. In order to encompass these healing phenomena, we are compelled to describe yet another era—Era III, or the era of *nonlocal* medicine.

Era III

Era III medicine is the first form to make use of a genuinely nonlocal approach to the relationship of mind, body, and time. That is, it does not regard the mind as localized within an individual human brain or body, or confined to the present moment. In the Era III view, rather, minds are viewed as spread through space and time. One particular implication of this view is that human consciousness is unbounded—and if unbounded, then some aspect of the human psyche must ultimately be unified. As physicist Erwin Schrödinger put it, "Mind by its very nature is a *singulare tantum*. I should say: the overall number of minds is just one."[3]

The differences between Eras II and III are radical. Where Era II was solidly *local* in outlook, Era III is *nonlocal*, holding that the mind is unconfined to points in space or time. Era III also differs from Era II in regard to how it views the *nature* of the mind. For example, most people doing research in the area of mind-body medicine do not believe that they are witnessing the action of "mind" or "consciousness" on the body, but the action of *brain* on the body. The emphasis is not on what "consciousness" can do, but on what the brain can do. From this perspective Era II could be considered the era of "*brain*-body" medicine, not "*mind*-body" medicine. Some Era II researchers are very explicit in equating mind and brain. They would agree in principle with the point of view expressed by astronomer Carl Sagan, who said, "[The brain's] workings—what we sometimes call mind—are a consequence of its anatomy and physiology, and nothing more."[4]

The anomalous healing events that one sees in the Era II or mind-body area are generally regarded as only temporarily unexplainable. Most people believe that "when we know enough," we will be able to explain them in the familiar Newtonian framework. Thus we can call these events "low anomalies."

Low anomalies stand in contrast to various types of nonlocal events that characterize Era III. In these phenomena the mind seems to escape the confines of the individual brain and body, and on occasion appears to escape the present moment as well. These events can be called "high anomalies." *High anomalies seem to have no possibility, even in principle, of being explained in the local, physicalistic, reductionistic framework of Eras I and II.* Because they do not conform to our familiar constructions of reality, they cause immense intellectual indigestion in medical science and are commonly dismissed as the results of poor observation, mistaken interpretation, or outright fraudulent reporting.

Why should medicine be concerned about "high anomalies"? The reason is straightforward: these events can and do affect the body in dramatic ways. I suggest that *anything* that significantly affects the functions of the body—whether it is a bacterium or virus, a drug or a surgical procedure, or a prayer—is the legitimate concern of medicine.

NONLOCAL MEDICAL EVENTS

Prayer-related healing, which is the focus of this book, is a genuinely Era III therapy. Why nonlocal? After much research I have been unable to find a single authority who will claim that the degree of spatial separation of the praying person from the subject is a factor in its effectiveness. Those who practice healing with prayer claim uniformly that these effects do not diminish with distance; prayer is as effective from the other side of the world as it is from next door or at the bedside. Such claims do not rest on anecdote or single-case studies. As we shall see when we examine the scientific evidence for prayer-type healing, numerous controlled studies have validated the nonlocal nature of prayer. Much of this evidence, moreover, suggests that praying individuals—or people involved in compassionate imagery or mental intent, whether or not it is called prayer—can purposefully affect the physiology of distant people without the "receiver's" awareness.

Prayer is only one of the many nonlocal phenomena to have healing implications. Before we examine more fully the evidence for its effectiveness, let's take a look at some of these other events. They will show us that a great variety of related happenings share a nonlocal character.

Diagnosis at a Distance

A remarkable example of the ability of the mind to manifest nonlocally in medically helpful ways is in long-distance, "intuitive" diagnosis. Perhaps the most persuasive example of this phenomenon is described in *The Creation of Health: Merging Medicine with Intuitive Diagnosis* by C. Norman Shealy, M.D., and Caroline M. Myss.[5]

In 1985 Dr. Shealy, a Harvard-trained neurosurgeon and researcher who founded the American Holistic Medical Association, met and began to work with Caroline Myss, a journalist who had no formal training in medicine or health. Since early childhood, however, she had had an intuitive ability to "know" things. Dr. Shealy asked her to put her intuitive skills to work in diagnosing illness in his patients. With a patient in his office in Missouri, he would phone Myss in New Hampshire, some twelve hundred miles away. Initially he would simply give her his patient's name and birth date, and she would then tell him her impressions. Most of these dealt with the patient's psychological conflicts. But as their partnership evolved, Shealy encouraged her to be as specific as possible about physical abnormalities. Then Myss began to "enter" the patient's body intuitively, as if she were the actual patient. Shealy encouraged her to travel through the patient's body systematically, examining the relative health of each organ system. According to Shealy's data, Myss is 93 percent accurate—"a fantastic accomplishment."[6] That is an understatement. Even with sophisticated diagnostic tools such as blood analyses and X rays, medical diagnosticians seldom achieve these levels of accuracy in the earliest phase of diagnosis.

At first Myss was hesitant to become involved with intuitive diagnosis. She had always considered her talent as a curiosity, something she could dabble in at will. She was particularly leery of labels such as "psychic," and was concerned about being thought fraudulent or "crackpot."

The geographical distance separating Myss and the patient is apparently overcome totally in the intuitive process. Myss feels that this distancing creates an impersonality that is important to her success because it permits her to "receive information that a more personal connection would otherwise tend to block."

Shealy cites fifty examples of Myss's intuitive diagnoses, most of which correspond with great accuracy to Shealy's actual medical diagnoses. As examples, when Myss diagnosed "migraine headache, myofascial pain," Shealy's diagnosis was "migraine headache, myofascial pain." Her "chest pain due to trauma" corresponded to his "post-surgical chest pain, left." Her "malignancy of [the] brain" was his "metastatic brain cancer," and so on. Shealy's estimation of Myss's skills is unequivocal: "I have not seen anyone more accurate than Caroline," he says, "not even a physician!"

Shealy sometimes knew the correct diagnosis at the time he contacted Myss. This has prompted some people to propose that he "telepathically transmitted" the information to her, and that she therefore did not make the diagnosis independently. This cannot be the whole story, because Myss *has* made correct diagnoses before they were known to anyone. And even if telepathy were involved in some cases, it, too, is an example of a nonlocal mental event and hardly less remarkable than diagnosis at a distance.

Does anything in the history of medical practice correspond to Myss's abilities? Perhaps. During the first half of the nineteenth century, the cult of "snap diagnosis" was the rage on the European continent. Physicians in the great teaching academies vied with each other to rattle off a correct diagnosis with as few clues as possible. A physician who was really good at this did not even need to see or examine the patient. Jean-Nicolas Corvisart, Napoleon's favorite physician, was allegedly one of the best. He once remarked that the subject of an oil painting must have been a victim of heart disease, and it proved to be so. The legendary physicians Hebra and Bell, for whom Bell's palsy is named, "could detect the occupations as well as the diseases of their patients."[7] The resemblance of the art of snap diagnosis to clairvoyance hardly needs mentioning.[8]

Seemingly exotic skills such as these may still be with us, and may be more common than we think. In a research project at a major medical school, computers were programmed to interview patients and diagnose their illnesses; their results were compared to the diagnoses of a group of skilled internists. Both the computer and physicians asked the patients identical questions, and the patients gave identical responses to both. The computer, however, was not nearly as successful as the doctors in making accurate diagnoses, a fact that puzzled the researchers. So they asked the internists, "What is the first thing you notice when you begin to interview the patient?" The internists replied, "Whether or not the patient looks sick." But the researchers could not determine precisely what "looks sick" meant, and they could find no way to program "looks sick" into the computer. The research project was abandoned. Any skilled diagnostician, however, knows what it means. It is a sense, an intuition, a difficult-to-describe "way of knowing" that bypasses the yes-and-no answers the patient gives, and may have nothing to do with actually seeing the patient. It may, as in Myss's case, operate independently of any sensory input at all from the patient.

Noncontact Therapeutic Touch

Since antiquity there have been people who have claimed the ability to heal from a distance, healers for whom the degree of spatial separation from the patient is reputed to be inconsequential. Also ancient is the practice of "laying on of hands," in which actual physical contact takes place between healer and healee. A hybridization of these techniques has recently taken place in professional nursing circles through the landmark research of nursing academician Dolores Krieger, Ph.D., of New York University.[9] In this technique, called Therapeutic Touch, the healer's hands do not actually touch the patient but are held a short distance from the patient's body.

To evaluate this technique, researcher Daniel P. Wirth performed a double-blind study involving forty-four patients with artificially created, full-skin-thickness surgical wounds. The subjects would insert the arm with the wound through a circular cut-out aperture in the wall of the facility, beyond which they could not see, for five minutes. They were told that the purpose of this procedure was to measure "biopotentials" from the surgical site with a noncontact device. A noncontact Therapeutic Touch practitioner was present in the adjoining room only during exposure sessions for members of the active treatment group (twenty-three patients); the room was vacant during the sham procedure periods for the remaining twenty-one patients. As she attempted to heal the wounds, the practitioner meticulously avoided any physical contact with the subjects. At several stages the wound area was traced on transparent acetate sheets by a physician "blinded" to patient assignment to active or sham groups; and then an independent technician, also blinded to the two groups, would digitize the tracings—an extremely accurate measurement of healing. It is important to remember that since the subjects did not *believe* they were receiving a healing treatment, and since they received neither overt nor covert suggestions of being participants in a healing experiment, the placebo response, suggestion, expectation, or belief cannot be held responsible for the healing that occurred.

The results were highly significant statistically. By day eight the wound sizes of the treated subjects showed much less variation than those of the untreated subjects, and were significantly smaller. On day sixteen this finding was again seen. Thirteen of the twenty-three treated subjects were completely healed (wound size zero), compared with *none* of the untreated group. This study indicated that noncontact Therapeutic Touch is an effective healing modality on full-thickness human dermal wounds, even if the subject is unaware of its occurrence.[10]

Is this a genuine Era III technique? If the healing influence of Therapeutic Touch practitioners depends on conventional forms of energy, we would expect the effect to deteriorate with increasing spatial separation of healer and healee because, according to the inverse square law, all known forms of energy weaken at a distance. Noncontact Therapeutic Touch would therefore only operate locally, not nonlocally, and to be most effective, the healer would need to be on site. Definitive studies have not yet been done to clarify this point. Until they are it may be stretching the point to classify noncontact Therapeutic Touch as an Era III method.[11]

Transpersonal Imagery

In her book *Imagery in Healing*, psychophysiologist-author Jeanne Achterberg advanced the idea that there are two kinds of mental imagery.[12] The first type, *preverbal* imagery, acts upon one's own physical being to change its physiological activity. The second type is what she calls *transpersonal* imagery, in which the consciousness of one person can affect the physical substrate of another. These two types of imagery correspond to what we have been calling local versus nonlocal types of events. They also fall within, respectively, the Era II (local, mind-body) and Era III (nonlocal) healing methodologies described above.

At the Mind Science Foundation in San Antonio, Texas, researchers William G. Braud and Marilyn Schlitz put nonlocal, transpersonal imagery to a test. They examined whether or not a person could use specific mental imagery to change the physical reactions of a distant person with whom they had no physical or sensory contact. They performed thirteen experiments using this strategy, and found a significant relationship between the use of calming or activating imagery of one person and the electrodermal activity of another isolated, distant subject (electrodermal activity is an indicator of physiological arousal). "The findings," the researchers stated, "demonstrate reliable and relatively robust anomalous interactions between living systems at a distance."[13] We will discuss these experiments more fully later.

Remote Sensing

For about a decade, studies done at Princeton University's Engineering Anomalies Research Laboratory (PEAR Lab) have indicated that subjects can influence the outcome of random physical events and can mentally convey complex information to other subjects from whom they are widely separated, even by global distances. These studies show not only that a sender can mentally transmit detailed information to a receiver on the other side of the earth, but also that the receiver usually "gets" the information up to three days *before* it is sent. The details of these studies are contained in Robert G. Jahn's and

Brenda J. Dunne's epochal book *Margins of Reality*.[14] These experiments demonstrate that the mind is nonlocal not only in *space* but in *time* as well.

Telesomatic Events

The vital force is not enclosed in man, but radiates around him like a luminous sphere, and it may be made to act at a distance. In these semimaterial rays the imagination of a man may produce healthy or morbid effects.

—Paracelsus (1493–1541)[15]

Research in the field of psychosomatic medicine has demonstrated beyond reasonable doubt that disturbances in the mind can cause bodily dysfunction and disease *within* an individual—the Era II or mind-body perspective described above. But if mind is nonlocal and thus shared, the possibility arises that mental events can trigger happenings *between* individuals as well. These phenomena have been called "telesomatic"—from the Greek *tele*, meaning "far off," and *somatikos*, referring to "body."[16] Examples are legion:

• Arthur Severn, a well-known British landscape painter, went out for an early morning sail while his wife was still asleep. She was suddenly awakened at about 7:00 A.M. by a blow to her lip, which was so violent she immediately began to look for blood. To her surprise she found none. Later in the morning, when her husband returned for breakfast, he was holding a handkerchief to his bleeding lips—having been hit in the mouth at about 7:00 A.M., when the boat's tiller swung in a gust of wind.[17]

• A woman suddenly "doubled over, clutching her chest as if in severe pain, and said, 'Something has happened to Nell, she has been hurt.'" Two hours later the sheriff came, stating that Nell had died on the way to the hospital. She had been involved in an auto accident, in which a piece of the steering wheel had penetrated her chest.[18]

• A mother was writing a letter to her daughter, who was away at college. Suddenly her right hand started to burn so severely she couldn't hold the pen. Less than an hour later, she received a phone call from the college telling her that her daughter's right hand had been severely burned by acid in a laboratory accident, at the same time she (the mother) had felt the burn.[19]

• Sometimes actual physical changes appear in the "receiver." In 1892 British Major-General T. Blaksley reported a case involving a close soldier-friend in the 12th Regiment who felt unaccountably ill one morning. On their way to the firing ranges his friend said, on the basis of sheer intuition, "My twin brother died this morning on his ship on the West coast of Africa, at eight o'clock, and I know that the effect on me will be a serious illness." General Blaksley tried to raise his hopes by persuading the man he had been dreaming, but to no avail. "No," his friend insisted, "it is certain; through our lives there has always been such strong sympathy between us that nothing has ever happened to one without the other knowing about it." His presentiments proved correct. He came down with an attack of jaundice. The news came in due course that his brother had indeed died at the time he had stated.[20]

Skeptics will, of course, find nothing meaningful in events of this sort. They will claim that they are nothing more than mere coincidences. It is true that these events are anecdotes. One cannot compel them to happen in the laboratory so they can be studied under close scrutiny. They are unlike other nonlocal events we've examined—transpersonal imagery, distant diagnosis, and remote sensing—that *can* be studied under controlled conditions. In spite of these limitations, however, I believe telesomatic events deserve our attention for two reasons. First, they are extraordinarily commonplace. Second, they exhibit an internal consistency from case to case. Almost all of them happen between people who are *empathic*—a feeling that, as we shall see, seems to set the stage for nonlocal events in the laboratory. Telesomatic events commonly occur between individuals with strong emotional bonds. The classic case involves parents and children. They are also characteristic between spouses, siblings (particularly identical twins), and lovers, but have been described also between friends and acquaintances who are emotionally close.[21]

Telesomatic events frequently convey information of life-or-death importance. Everyone has heard of a mother who "just knows" her child is in peril and rushes home to drag the daughter from the swimming pool just in time. These occurrences manifest in other ways that can be medically important. For example, a fifty-six-year-old woman, who had stopped menstrual bleeding eight years earlier, had three episodes of uterine bleeding at the same time that one of her daughters experienced unexpected labor and the other threatened to have an abortion. The daughters were living miles away, and she was completely uninformed about their respective conditions. Twenty months later the woman had a massive uterine hemorrhage, at which point she was found to have a cancer of the lining of the uterus, which may have increased the likelihood that she would bleed from this part of the body in concert with her daughters.[22]

In her analysis of 169 telesomatic cases, Louisa E. Rhine found that only two receivers were husbands, compared to twenty-one instances in which the receivers were wives. Moreover, out of the total 169 cases, only thirteen of the receiving people were male.[23] But other series' findings do not support such gender differences. In Stevenson's sample, for instance, eighty-four receivers were female and seventy-six male. In contrast sixty-two of the "senders" were female and ninety-eight male.[24]

Are women more sensitive receivers than men? Or do they simply report their experiences more freely? Stevenson, whose data were fairly gender neutral, does believe that gender differences are real, that women may have a greater tendency to be in touch paranormally with members of the opposite sex.

The higher incidence of women as receivers fits with the common impression by physicians that psychosomatic symptoms are more frequent in women. All too often physicians make this observation in a pejorative way, as if psychosomatic susceptibility is a weakness. Not surprisingly this opinion has been criticized as being "sexist" and biased—just what one would expect, many say, from a male-dominated profession. But rather than being a weakness, the increased sensitivity of women in receiving the experiences of distant people may reflect a psychological and perhaps biological superiority. Of course one must factor in the fact that women are acculturated to "be sensitive." These same cultural pressures may inhibit men's receptivity to the distant experiences of others. Further study would have to be done before any firm conclusions could be drawn about gender and telesomatics.

There can be surprising pressure even from within organized religions to suppress spontaneous experiences of this sort. In a letter written from Toledo to Don Lorenzo de Cepeda in January 1577, St. Teresa of Avila said, "I've had raptures again. They're most embarrassing. Several times in public . . . during Matins, for instance. I'm so ashamed, I simply want to hide away somewhere!"[25] In some traditions, such as Zen Buddhism, these types of experiences are not suppressed but simply are not encouraged, because it is felt they can be a potential distraction from more important spiritual work. For example, "[A] Zen master . . . after listening to one of his students report on the vision of Light and True Buddhahood that he had experienced during meditation, responded soberly, 'Keep meditating. It will go away.' "[26] Or as Suzuki Roshi said, "What do you want to get enlightened for? You may not like it."[27]

While the telesomatic pathway appears to operate commonly between two people, several parties are sometimes involved, as in a case in which a woman had the distinct impression that her mother was seriously ill and needed her. Against the protests of her husband, she struck out to see her mother, only to meet her sister as she approached the mother's house. The sister had had the same impression and was similarly acting on it. Both women found their mother dying, asking for her daughters.[28]

A sense of empathy or emotional closeness appears to underlie many nonlocal events. This "heart connection" between subjects underlies transpersonal imagery, telesomatic events, and prayer-type healing, and it also appears to be a factor in human-machine interactions, as we shall see. This internal consistency is striking, and internal consistency is a quality highly prized in scientific investigation. If scientists can identify a "pattern that connects," a common thread tying together events that on the surface seem unrelated, this increases the scientific respectability of the events being studied and makes them appear "more real." In the next chapter we'll take a closer look at the role of prayer in healing, and the factors that influence its efficacy.

PART 2

FACTORS INFLUENCING
THE EFFICACY OF PRAYER

Chapter 3

Prayer and the Unconscious Mind

Seek not abroad,
turn back into thyself
for in the inner man dwells the truth.

—St. Augustine (A.D. 400), *City of God*

Every major religion has referred to inner guidance in its
teachings . . . the Spirit of Christ, the Atman, God within
. . .

—Christine M. Comstock

Carol was one of the healthiest patients I had ever had. She never came to see me except for routine exams, which were few and far between. Like many people interested in a holistic approach, Carol prided herself on "taking full responsibility" for her health and for "consciously creating [her] own reality"—100 percent!

One night at 3:00 A.M., I was called to the emergency room. There lay Carol on a stretcher, barely conscious and near death. Her blood pressure was dangerously low and she had a temperature of 105 degrees Fahrenheit. Her abdomen was rigid and tender, indicating some type of intra-abdominal catastrophe. After a few tests, she was taken to surgery, where she was successfully operated on for a ruptured appendix.

A few days later, I went by her hospital room to ask her specifically about the events leading up to her brush with death. Appendicitis usually gives plenty of warning signs—hours or days of pain, fever, nausea, and so on. "Carol, you must have known something was wrong. Why didn't you call me or come in to the office?"

Immediately she began to sob. Finally she managed to say through her tears, "Because I was so ashamed! I felt like a complete failure!" Carol's heroic task of fashioning her reality through her conscious efforts had failed. Her world had crumbled and lay in shambles all about her.[1]

Carol's case is not rare. David Spiegel, professor of psychiatry and behavioral sciences and director of the Psychosocial Treatment Laboratory at Stanford University School of Medicine, has reported similar cases:

> [A] woman in our [cancer support] group, a brilliant woman who wrote books on computer programming, had . . . gone to get special training in visualization techniques. When she came back and learned that her disease had spread substantially, she called a counselor from the imagery group, who said to her, "Why did you want your cancer to spread?" Fortunately, she was strong enough to tell him to go to hell. But many patients are afflicted with this burden of guilt, that if you can't control the course of disease, it must be your fault.[2]

Patients sometimes become so enamored with "self-responsibility" and "total personal control" that they are willing to carry these concepts to extremes. They may totally abandon conventional approaches, even in life-or-death situations. Another of Spiegel's cases:

> A woman in our [psychological support] group was also attending a group in which she visualized her cancer cells being eaten by her leukocyte [white blood] cells. She decided not only to drop out of our group but also to stop receiving chemotherapy and radiation. We argued vigorously with her not to do that. I said, "If you want to visualize, visualize, but stay with your medical treatment." She quit anyway, and she was dead within a year.[3]

Today increasing numbers of people are striving, like Carol, to use consciousness in the task of remaining healthy or getting well, of creating their own health-realities, and of claiming full responsibility for everything that happens. These efforts frequently involve prayer—either praying for oneself or enlisting the prayers of others. Enthusiasts, including believers in prayer, seem largely to deny the obvious: As we've seen already, no approach works 100 percent of the time—not prayer, not imagery, not visualization, or any other holistic approach that emphasizes self-reliance; not surgery, radiation, or the most potent "miracle" drugs. To rely on a single approach, no matter how philosophically or metaphysically attractive it might be, is to court disaster. Advocates all too often ignore these potential difficulties. They imply that prayer, positive thinking, and mental effort can only help the person using them, or that they will simply be ineffective. But there is a growing body of evidence that they can actually be harmful. "Positive thinking" has side effects, and the "force-feeding of hope" is being increasingly criticized as dangerous.[4]

Is this a contradiction? This book, after all, *emphasizes* self-responsibility and reliance on alternative methods of healing, including prayer. There is no contradiction. All techniques can be used unwisely. One of the pitfalls in their use is a confusion over what we mean by "consciousness."

WHAT IS "CONSCIOUSNESS"?

When someone speaks of their "consciousness" today—as in when they claim that they are using their consciousness to create their own health reality—they are almost invariably referring to the part of the mind that is *aware*. One of the practically unchallenged facts of modern psychology, however, is that we live the vast bulk of our psychic lives *not* in awareness but in *un*awareness or *un*consciousness.[5] This presents an immediate problem. If we are not even aware of the larger part of our psyche and what it may be doing, how then can we claim total, conscious responsibility for what happens in our life, including our health?

It is extremely odd that the role of the unconscious almost never comes up when people talk about the place of the mind in health. Particularly in religious circles, there seems a virtual embargo on acknowledging the unconscious mind. Why are we reluctant to talk about our unconscious? Why do we behave as if it doesn't exist? Why do we pretend that everything is "out front" in awareness, when overwhelming evidence tells us this simply is not so?

Perhaps it is because we don't trust the unconscious. Many people see it as a sinister force that pushes them around against their will—a dark repository of unacceptable, unflattering thoughts and emotions such as lust, hatred, and greed. Sigmund Freud, the chief architect of psychoanalysis, is largely responsible for this picture. Freud believed the unconscious could not be trusted. He maintained that the unconscious is the region of the id, a domain of psychic forces compelling us, among other things, to hate our mother or father, to have incestual desires and homicidal thoughts, and to indulge in unacceptable fantasies and wishes. The goal of therapy for Freud was to bring as many of these unconscious drives into awareness as possible, or to keep the lid on them through the use of socially acceptable psychological defense mechanisms.

Other explorers of the psyche saw the unconscious quite differently. Jung, for instance, conceived of a spectrum existing in the unconscious: the layers closest to our awareness are more or less capable of becoming known; those farthest away are in principle inaccessible to our awareness and operate autonomously. Jung saw the unconscious as the home of timeless psychic forces he called archetypes, which generally are invariant throughout all cultures and eras. He felt that every psychic force has its opposite in the unconscious—the force of light is always counterposed with that of darkness, good with evil, love with hate, life with death, on and on. Jung believed that *any* psychic energy could get out of hand and become unbalanced. *There could even be too much harmony and goodness* in human beings. It is the nature of the deep archetypal forces always to strive for balance between opposing qualities of all types. The goal of a lifetime, Jung maintained, is to achieve a dynamic balance of the innate opposites and to make this balancing process as conscious as possible.

We will never be able to take full advantage of the power of the mind to shape our health—including the mind's use of prayer—until we broaden our concept of "consciousness." This means including the unconscious and acknowledging that it is more than the hangout of the bogeymen and monsters we generally think it to be. If we do so, we shall see that the unconscious can be extraordinarily helpful and benevolent in our quest for health. In fact *the unconscious mind can initiate or cooperate with prayer and even mediate the effects.*

But we should prepare ourselves for surprises. Even though the unconscious may strive mightily to ensure our survival during moments of crisis such as grave illness, it does so on its own terms. It will even violate the values we hold dearest in our aware, conscious life, such as our moral and ethical codes, in order to help us. It will employ devices that, during our waking moments, we would almost always reject. Let's look at some examples.

Denial in the Coronary Care Unit

The most effective psychological coping strategy in the acute phase of a heart attack, after one is in the coronary care unit (CCU), is *denial*.[6] (I must caution that *before* one reaches the hospital, denial can be dangerous and even fatal, because it can cause one to delay seeking medical care. In fact denial is one of the reasons why 60 percent of patients with acute heart attacks die before reaching a treatment facility.[7]) Genuine denial wells up from the unconscious. It is highly irrational and illogical; it flies in the face of obvious facts. A physician may say to a patient who is lying in the CCU, "Joe, you've had a heart attack, no doubt about it. Your symptoms and physical examination are typical, your electrocardiogram clearly shows the damage, and your blood tests are positive—the most classic heart attack I've ever seen." Joe listens impassively and then says, "I appreciate your concern, Doctor, but this is just muscle pain or indigestion. I'm too young; nobody in my family has ever had a heart attack at this age. Besides, I really don't have time for this. I've got a busy schedule at the office. Look, I need to be out of here in a couple of hours." Even though this response is irrational, studies have shown that people who use it survive in greater numbers than those who confront the facts squarely and honestly. In fact no other psychological coping style is correlated with such a high survival rate in the acute phase of a myocardial infarction.

This can pose problems for people who are praying that Joe will survive his heart attack. They might say, "I wanted my prayer to work, but not *that* way! I didn't want Joe to start lying to himself!"

How does denial work? Researchers believe it allays anxiety because the patient doesn't believe the heart attack is real. This in turn leads to lower blood levels of adrenaline, a calmer blood pressure and heart rate, and a decreased susceptibility to life-threatening irregularities of the heartbeat. Thus the unconscious seems to set in motion through denial a pattern of physical responses tailor-made for survival.

Denial also has been shown to have life-saving value for certain people with breast cancer. In one research study, some of the women expressed denial of their illness in shocking ways: "I don't really have breast cancer," they said. "My doctor removed both my breasts and gave me chemotherapy and radiation because he wanted to be very careful; he didn't want to take any chances." Those women who responded to their initial diagnosis with brazen denial had practically the same survival statistics over a ten-year period as those who faced up to their diagnoses with openness and honesty.[8]

I have discovered that people don't like to hear these stories. Such accounts challenge their hallowed ideas about "taking responsibility" and being the sole, purposeful, *conscious* creator of their medical reality. But this data will not go away, and it poses great challenges to how we view the role of the unconscious mind in our health.

"Don't Relax, Be Worried"

Almost everyone is afraid before undergoing major surgery. We fear giving up all control during anesthesia, being suspended helplessly between life and death, being opened up surgically, and so on. Many of these anxieties are lodged in the unconscious. Try as we may, we cannot shut them out. They emerge in dreams, in nightmares, and in our waking life. They erupt unexpectedly in those quiet interludes when the conscious mind lets its guard down; they gnaw at us when we're not even thinking about surgery. Psychologists tell us it's best to acknowledge these apprehensions and bring them into total awareness so they can be dealt with and laid to rest before having surgery, and there is a virtual growth industry of therapists who teach people how to do this.

British psychologist Anne Manyande of University College in London and her colleagues examined blood levels of two stress hormones, adrenaline and cortisol, in patients just before surgery, in the recovery room, and on the two days following surgery.[9] These stress hormones are believed to contribute to weight loss, fatigue, and impaired immune function surrounding major surgery. They found that the stress hormone levels increased significantly only in those patients who were given relaxation training for their anxieties and fears prior to surgery. In patients not taught coping strategies, the hormone levels remained normal. The relaxation training did work in other ways: patients receiving it reported less anxiety and worry, had a lower heart rate and blood pressure, and required fewer pain-killing drugs following surgery.

Peter Salmon, one of the researchers, believes that relaxation training may distract people from focusing constructively on their upcoming surgery. "Our hypothesis is that thinking about and preparing for a stressful event is a better tactic," he says.[10] Wipe out all the noxious feelings and emotions, and the incentive to plan ahead can be thrown off track. Abolish all the worries, and we may stop thinking of ways to deal with pain and immobility, what the illness means, how best to manage our life during the period of sickness and recuperation, and so on. The body seemingly *needs* a bit of worry and fear before surgery, and our unconscious mind seems to know this fully.

This study does not stand alone. At the University of Cincinnati Medical School, researchers have found that the pregnant woman who has anxiety-ridden and threatening dream images about her baby and her approaching labor usually experiences a shorter and easier labor than the woman whose dreams are full of happier, more pleasant images. Surveying these findings, dream researchers Jayne Gackenbach and Jane Bosveld say, "It's as if the threatening dreams are acknowledging the painful event that is to come, while the more pleasant dreams deny that reality just as perhaps the woman who is dreaming them is denying the pain that will be sure to accompany birth."[11]

You Create My Reality, I Create Yours

One of the propositions of this book is that *other people* can participate in creating our health reality, and that we can participate in creating theirs. This is an unavoidable implication of intercessory prayer, demonstrated in the various laboratory experiments examined in Appendix 1. This possibility is also strongly supported by research in transpersonal imagery at the Mind Science Foundation in San Antonio,

Texas. In a series of exemplary experiments, Dr. William G. Braud and his colleagues have shown that the mental images of one person can modify the activity of the autonomic nervous system of a distant person, even when the "receiver" is unaware that the attempt is being made.[12]

As we shall see throughout this book, this evidence points to the existence of a profoundly *nonlocal* aspect of the psyche—some quality of the mind that is not confined to points in space such as brains or bodies, or to points in time such as the present moment. This evidence simply cannot be ignored, and it plays havoc with the notion that my conscious "I" is the sole architect of my medical reality.

LETTING GO

Attempting to use only the consciously aware part of the mind is like trying to shoot an arrow by pushing it forward from the bow string. Everyone knows it's best to pull the string back and let the power of the bow do the work. In many situations one has to *let go* in the realization that there simply are some things one cannot *make* happen. Relying on the hidden, unseen power of our unconscious mind is like that.

How can we do this? The first step is to acknowledge that the inner, unseen, unconscious part of the mind comprises most of the human psyche and that, try as we might, it is *impossible in principle* to be completely aware of this dimension of the psyche. The next step is to honor the capacity of the unconscious to come to our need in extremely potent ways. Next, we might try simply to *make friends* with our unconscious—to cease to mistrust it.

The value of this approach is nowhere more apparent than in so-called miracle cures. The late Brendan O'Regan, who was vice president for research at the Institute of Noetic Sciences in Sausalito, California, studied these phenomena extensively, and concluded that people undergoing radical, spontaneous healing events "are in a different place psychologically." One of their chief characteristics is that they do not determinedly want healing; they are not desperate for a miracle to occur; they are not trying at any cost to extract a radical healing from the universe. They have a quality of acceptance and gratitude, as if things are quite all right in spite of the presence of the disease. Thus the paradox: those who do not demand healing are the ones who frequently seem to receive it. When asked what they did to bring about the healing, they reply, "I didn't *do* anything. It 'just happened.'"[13]

Learning "how to be" can set in motion not only healing but the power *to* heal. A dramatic example occurred in the life of Alvar Nuñez Cabeza de Vaca, the Spanish explorer who followed the wake of Columbus to the New World during the first half of the sixteenth century. After becoming shipwrecked and stranded on the Texas coast, de Vaca feared murder by hostile natives. He and two fellow survivors dug a pit, where they spent several cold winter nights sleeping naked. De Vaca and his colleagues had lost everything—yet they not only survived, but underwent an amazing transformation: they emerged from the pit with the power to heal. On their way westward, their fame spread ahead of them. The natives would bring their sick, and de Vaca and his friends would heal them, and they were thus able to travel unharmed. Eventually they made their way back to Mexico City, the seat of Spanish civilization in the New World.[14]

De Vaca's ability to heal was preceded by a profound emptiness, a shipwreck of both body and spirit, a dark night of the soul in which he did not know if he would survive. A miracle was born not out of his *doing*, but from the unconscious depths of his *being*.

Five centuries later a similar event took place in one of the most hostile regions on earth: Antarctica. In July 1989, six men, each from a different nation, began the first unmechanized trek across the Antarctic continent. This remarkable effort, known as the International Trans-Antarctica Expedition, was led by former science teacher Will Steger of the United States, who previously had led an expedition without resupply to the North Pole in 1986. For 220 days the group braved the worst weather in the world, enduring two months of storms, winds up to ninety miles an hour, and temperatures as low as minus 43 degrees Fahrenheit. By dog sled and skis, following the longest and most difficult route across Antarctica, they completed their goal 3,741 miles later.

Just two days before the completion of their journey a blinding snowstorm arose. At 4:30 in the afternoon, thirty-two-year-old Keizo Funatsu of Japan, the youngest member of the expedition and the team's expert with sled dogs, walked a few yards from the camp in the blizzard to feed the huskies. Although the men had staked skis and poles every few yards between their tents, a common precaution in such conditions, Funatsu lost his way. Realizing his precarious situation, he took immediate measures for survival. This is how he later described his experience in his journal:

> Once I was in my snow ditch, blowing snow covered me in five, ten seconds. . . . I could breathe through a cavity close to my body. . . . I knew my teammates would be looking for me. I believed I would be found. . . . I said to myself, "Settle down, try and enjoy this." In my snow ditch I truly felt Antarctica. With the snow and quiet covering me, I felt like I was in my mother's womb. I could hear my heart beat—boom, boom, boom—like a small baby's. My life seemed very small compared to nature, to Antarctica.

Two hours after Funatsu became lost in the white-out conditions, the other team members discovered his absence and began a four-hour search, which had to be abandoned because of darkness and the storm. At 4:00 A.M. the next day, they resumed. At 6:00 A.M. Funatsu, unhurt, heard the searchers calling his name. He emerged from his snowy thirteen-and-a-half hour burial and stood up, shouting, "I am alive! I am alive!"[15]

Completely covered with snow, Funatsu realized that to *do* anything would have meant almost certain death. He had simply to *be*. The images that flooded his mind were those of the most profound period of not-doing for anyone—being a baby in his mother's womb. Thus buried alive at the bottom of the world, he could only wait patiently to see what the universe would deliver. His "being strategy"—his not-doing, his receptivity—paid off with survival, as it did for de Vaca.[16]

Some people would respond to this point of view by saying, "You are asking us to be completely passive, to give up, to ignore our own efforts to improve our health. You're saying it doesn't make any difference what we consciously think—that it's all in the hands of the unconscious or of others who may be shaping what happens to us outside our knowledge. You want us to abandon all personal control and responsibility for our health. You are even advocating using denial and the lying, scheming, and dishonesty that are part of it."

This is a misunderstanding, as anyone who has learned to tap the power of the unconscious mind knows. For one thing, relying on the power of the unconscious does not mean that we must abandon all voluntary effort. Neither does it mean we should forego surgery, medications, and other modern forms of intervention that can be decidedly helpful. We can and should continue to act as wisely as possible and take *appropriate* responsibility for our health. Neither does it mean that we have to be overly worried about the excessive use of denial. After all, denial contains a built-in safety feature. If we try to use it consciously, it ceases to be denial, for genuine denial wells up from the *un*conscious and is not elected from conscious choice.

Underlying the desire for total personal, conscious control and responsibility in health is frequently a narcissistic desire for power. While it is true that personal, conscious effort may seem to suffice as long as life is smooth, when major problems occur—as they almost always will, as in the case of Carol's ruptured appendix—this illusion of total self-sufficiency can be painfully shattered.

WE DON'T *CREATE* THE WORLD, WE *ARE* THE WORLD—100 PERCENT!

Philosopher Alan Watts once said that the sun would not be "bright" were it not for human eyes; thorns would not be "prickly" if skin were not soft; rocks would not be "hard" or "heavy" if muscles did not exist; and so on. "Bright," "prickly," "hard," and "heavy" are definable only by reference to our own senses. A century earlier Ralph Waldo Emerson arrived at the identical idea. We habitually attribute too much to the world, he observed, and not enough to ourselves. Emerson used the example of a rose, which for its "fragrance" and "color" depends on *us*. Physicist P. W. Bridgman recently arrived at a similar conclusion. As he put it, "In general we should never think of the world around us without also thinking of the nervous machinery in our heads by means of which we acquire knowledge of the world."[17]

Throughout human history, representatives from all the major spiritual traditions, both East *and* West, have glimpsed the realization described by Watts, Emerson, and Bridgman: that there is a deep and ineradicable reciprocity between the world and us, and that it makes no sense to separate existence into a dual subject and object. Zen Buddhism, for example, expresses this relationship in the philosophy of "dependent co-arising," in which all opposites are said to arise mutually and to define each other.

An increasing number of modern scientists appear to agree. For example, the developmental biologist R. Davenport has stated that we are capable of knowing something only because *differences* or *contrasts* arise. Because it takes at least two things to make a difference or to form a contrast, one of which is our own psyche, it follows that we are in some sense responsible for what we call "reality." Take away our psyche—which includes our unconscious as well as our conscious—and there is no experience, in which case all talk of "the world" and "reality" is purely speculative and hypothetical. As Davenport puts it,

> If we examine the experiences from which our knowledge of the world arises, we can see that they consist of various types of differences. Without difference, there can be no experience. The experience of difference is basic to our notion of existence, the latter being derived from the Latin *ex sistere*, which means "to stand apart," i.e., to be different. . . . [S]ince all properties must be experienced as difference, the physical world exists for us only in terms of relationships. . . . [P]hysical reality does not exist before us as an object of study but *emerges from our consciousness during our changing experience within nature.*"[18]

When wise teachers throughout history have spoken about "going beyond dualism," "giving up the ego," or "penetrating the opposites," they are sanctioning the same idea: We don't *observe* or *create* the world as if it were an object, we *are* in some sense that very world.

DREAM PRAYER

Pray without ceasing.

—1 Thessalonians 5:17 (KJV)

And he spake a parable unto them to this end, that men ought always to pray. . . .

—Luke 18:1 (KJV)

> But we will give ourselves continually to prayer.
>
> —Acts 6:4 (KJV)

> . . . [B]e constant in prayer.
>
> —Romans 12:12
>
> (Revised Standard Version [RSV])

The unconscious mind complicates prayer considerably. As we've seen it works toward health in ways that may oppose the wishes of conscious awareness. If we pray only for what is acceptable to the latter—for less pain, fear, and anxiety—we may be violating the wishes of the unconscious and its potent healing effects. When we pray, therefore, we ought always to bear in mind the desires of the unconscious. But if they are indeed unconscious, how can we know them? One of the best ways is to pay attention to dreams.

As a child one of the most puzzling pieces of advice I ever heard shouted from the pulpit was the exhortation to "pray unceasing." I was old enough to realize that "unceasing" meant "nonstop," and I tried to comply with this biblical imperative night after night. I would lie silently in bed, fighting sleep with every ounce of determination I could muster as I said my prayers over and over to myself. But try as I might, I simply was not capable of nonstop prayer. I would always succumb to sleep's tug and resume my prayers in the morning.

I was immensely puzzled how any human being could conceivably pray continually. To be able to do so, I reasoned that they would have to be able to pray in their sleep, and I recall wondering if it were possible to pray during one's dreams. I was much attracted to this possibility, as it seemed infinitely less painful than waking prayer.

I had no idea, of course, that certain people throughout history have indeed believed that "dream prayer" is possible. In his book *Prayer: Finding the Heart's True Home*, Richard J. Foster relates that Isaac the Syrian believed that one could "pray unceasing," even during sleep:

> When the Spirit has come to reside in someone, that person cannot stop praying; for the Spirit prays without ceasing in him. No matter if he is asleep or awake, prayer is going on in his heart all

the time. He may be eating or drinking, he may be resting or working—the incense of prayer will ascend spontaneously from his heart. The slightest stirring of his heart is like a voice which sings in silence and in secret to the Invisible.[19]

One who has attained this state is not so much praying as "being prayed," literally taken over by prayer. A state of prayerfulness has infiltrated not just the conscious mind but the unconscious as well, including sleep and dreams. Foster observes that St. Francis seemed to fit this description. He "seemed not so much a man praying as prayer itself made man."[20]

Today we equate prayer almost exclusively with waking awareness and rationality. It is something done consciously through the medium of language. That prayer might occur "out of sight, out of mind" in the depths of the unconscious, even during dreams, may seem preposterous. And the possibility that our unconscious might know how to pray better than our conscious mind is simply not entertained. *But why shouldn't prayer be part of the repertoire of the unconscious? Our unconscious comprises the vast majority of our mental life. If prayer is a valuable activity, should not the bulk of our psyche wish to participate in it?*

One of the bedrock tenets of Jung's psychology is that there is an intrinsic drive toward wholeness and integration within the psyche of all people. This "urge to oneness" is quintessentially spiritual. It underlies the visions of all great religious traditions—the need to return or somehow reconnect with the Absolute, God, Goddess, Tao, Brahman, Allah, however the Ultimate may be conceived. *This urge toward wholeness is the most elemental quality of prayer and prayerfulness*—the feeling that one is being drawn toward something higher, greater, deeper. In its most highly developed form, this feeling is expressed by mystics as the Divine Union or merging with the Absolute.

Jung maintained that something similar occurs in the unconscious during sleep and dreams. Over his lifetime he collected and analyzed thousands of instances in which the primordial urge toward wholeness emerged dramatically in recurring dream motifs—mandalas, images, natural symbols, and ineffable feelings that sometimes left the person feeling changed or transformed on waking.

If the urge toward oneness, unity, and wholeness lies at the heart of prayer—and if this urge erupts consistently during dreams when the unconscious takes the stage—we must consider seriously that prayer and dreaming are very closely related, and that we pray unconsciously night after night, dream after dream.

"Dream prayer" may indeed be our most effective prayer, because it occurs when the inhibitions and distractions of waking awareness and the ego have abated for a few hours. Unobstructed, the unconscious during sleep and dreams may be free to realize its natural, innate affinity with the Divine.

DREAMS OF WHOLENESS

In one of the best books on the subject of lucid dreams (dreams during which the dreamer knows he or she is dreaming), *Control Your Dreams*, Jayne Gackenbach and Jane Bosveld describe several dreams in which the dreamer experienced the mystical ideal of unity with the Divine.[21] Psychotherapist Kenneth Kelzer had a lucid dream he called the "Gift of the Magi," in which he was one of the three wise men searching for the infant Jesus. As he and his companions are traveling, "I enter a state of deep meditation and see so clearly that my ability to see the star at all is based on my inner attunement. Without this fine, delicate, inner tuning of consciousness I would not even see the star nor care that Christ had been born, much less find him." When Kelzer finally reaches the Christ child, he experiences a rush of emotion so intense he begins to cry, and his emotions about the meaning of the journey and finding the child flood him. He kneels on seeing the child, "entranced by the dazzling, beautiful light that emanates continuously from his whole body and especially from his loving eyes that simply look back at me, so calm and steady. . . . I feel as if I could kneel here forever." The effect lingered. Years later, Kelzer feels inspired whenever he thinks of the dream.

Gackenbach and Bosveld report a dream by Daryl Hewitt, a lucid dreamer who pursues spiritual experiences in his dreams. A meditator in his waking life, he began intentionally to allow himself to meditate during his lucid dreams out of a longing "for some greater depth and meaning." In one such dream, he begins to fly. Wanting to perceive things as deeply as possible, he actually begins to pray, saying, "Highest Father-Mother, help me to get the most from this." Shortly thereafter Hewitt began to experience

> potent flashes of extreme clarity—what seem to be glimpses of higher reality, in some way deeply personal and familiar. One of these flashes is accompanied by an image from afar of an Eastern spiritual master I admire. I feel convinced that these glimpses are indeed flashes of a higher reality, and can honestly say it is one of the most intensely spiritual experiences of my life.[22]

In lucid dreaming one knows that one is actually dreaming, and one can purposely use strategies to influence the content of the dream. If one wanted to pursue dreams of wholeness and a sense of oneness with the Absolute, what techniques could one use? At the California Institute of Integral Studies, Fariba Bogzaran conducted a study in which she asked a group of seventy-six volunteers, all of whom had lucid dreams, to "seek the highest" during their lucid dream moments. The ways they expressed this desire fell into two main categories. One group used a directed, specific approach—"I want to find God." Others were more nondirected and asked for no specific outcome—"Allow me to experience the Divine"—whatever that might mean. Bogzaran concluded that in the more passive seekers, the dream "seemed to be more profound," more powerful and enriching. As one dreamer put it, "I felt a renewed feeling of awe . . . respect for the splendor of the universe."[23]

Dreams of wholeness may erupt spontaneously and unannounced from the unconscious, but they clearly can be encouraged as well. This is an area where conscious intent, such as waking prayer and meditation, can synchronize with our unconscious processes, yielding immensely enriching experiences. Gackenbach and Bosveld make this clear.

> In order to be able to [experience the mystical dream], . . . one's desire must be a well-established ideal within the dreamer's mind. Without an idea to serve as a pattern, the experience lacks direction and can perhaps be confusing or harmful. . . . Preparation and direction . . . [guide] the mind toward new forms of conscious awareness including lucid dreams.[24]

DREAMS AND HEALING

One of the most common forms of prayer is for healing. If prayer and dreams are related, can dreams heal?

Psychologist Sandra Ingerman, who has pioneered a form of therapy called shamanic journeying, describes in her book *Welcome Home: Life After Healing* how prayer and dreams can come together for a cure when conventional approaches have failed. For years she endured a painful problem that medical specialists declared untreatable. Their only advice was that she get used to living with the pain. Desperate for a solution, Ingerman prayed every night before going to bed for help to come to her in a dream. Nothing happened until months later, when she dreamt one night that she was in her house when suddenly a young, handsome Native American appeared from behind her couch and declared that he had always lived there, only she did not know it. He was dressed in blue jeans and a blue work shirt, and held a rattle made of an extraordinary, translucent blue skin. He pointed to the place in her body where she experienced her pain and, after telling her she had a problem there, he shook his rattle over the area. At that moment she felt the pain leave her body and knew even while dreaming that she had experienced a cure. When she awakened, the pain was indeed gone; ten years hence, it has not returned. From that day forward, Ingerman has turned to her dreams for help in resolving both emotional and physical issues. Although the healing dream doesn't always come on the first try, it eventually arrives if she keeps asking. She also uses prayers and dreams as a therapeutic intervention with her clients. She frequently prays that a healing dream be sent to them, although never without their consent.[25]

Joseph, a professional writer from San Francisco, describes a healing dream involving his *typewriter*. It malfunctioned, and he scheduled a service appointment with a technician for the following day. That night the repairman appeared in Joseph's dream, told him he was sick and could not come, and gave specific instructions about how Joseph could make the necessary repairs himself. On waking, Joseph learned that the technician had indeed called in sick. With the instructions still fresh in his mind, he went to his typewriter, opened it, found the problem exactly as it appeared in the dream, and perfectly made the repairs.[26]

In *Imagery in Healing*, Jeanne Achterberg describes how sick people in ancient Greece would journey to a temple of healing, undergo ritual purification, and stay for the night in hopes of receiving healing while asleep.[27] This way of healing—a "nocturnal gift of a living god," as Gackenbach and Bosveld have called it—was also later engaged in by the Romans.[28]

We have examined one healing dream already—the famous case of St. Peregrine, whose cancer disappeared overnight in the wake of prayer and a dream that it would do so. But healing dreams are not just the stuff of antiquity, they are fairly common. For example, during a heated arm-wrestling match, David Pack of Knoxville, Tennessee, injured his arm. Despite six months of medical treatment, the pain and disability were so severe he had to leave his occupation in the construction business. Pack was desperate. One night, before falling asleep, he suggested to himself that his arm would be healed. "I recall a man in my dream state twisting and poking around on my elbow and it hurt," he said. "I asked him what he was doing, and he said, 'You have received two healings.'" On awakening Pack discovered that his right arm was tingling, just as if it had gone to sleep. But when the tingling left, so too had the pain, and his arm was "good as new." But what about the *two* healings mentioned by the "dream healer"? Later that week a cyst on his back burst—a problem that had been troubling him for ten years—finally relieving his chronic pain.[29]

INFLUENCE OF THE UNCONSCIOUS MIND ON OTHERS

Dreams of unity, wholeness, and healing can bring about healthy changes *within* our bodies, but can they affect the body of *someone else?* Can we pray successfully during our dreams for another? This a way of asking whether or not our individual unconscious mind can nonlocally "reach out" and affect a distant individual, who may be unaware we are trying to do so.

Some of the earliest investigations of the role of the unconscious mind in the transfer of information from one person to another were done in the Soviet Union in the early part of this century. Particularly interesting was the work in the 1920s of the Commission for the Study of Mental Suggestion, founded by V. M. Bekhterev.[30] In one series of experiments, a sender attempted to convey visual images to a receiver who was behind closed doors in a separate room. No physical or sensory contact took place between them. Before the experiment the sender chose three objects that were not in any way similar in shape, color, material composition, or utility. When the experiment began, he would look at only one of the three objects, examining its details, trying to focus solely on the object and bar any extraneous associations and thoughts from entering his mind. In spite of this, the visual imagery that entered the mind of the receiver usually had no appreciable similarity with the chosen object, but was filled with separate parts, details, or symbols of the object. For example, if the sender were focusing on the face of a pocket watch, the receiver perceived "a circle, a metal ring, a thought about figures, the image of an open compass, the hands of a watch, a working mechanism," and so on. Similarly, "Glass images usually elicited images of the surface of water or ice." In one experiment the sender's object was a brightly illuminated block of cut glass in the shape of a pyramidal polyhedron. The receiver saw "reflections in water—sugar loaf—snowy summit—iceberg, ice floes in the north illuminated by the sun—rays are broken up."

In another series of experiments, the sender drew a pair of scissors. The receiver responded, "I am plunging into something—a uniform with buttons and a cap—a bow tie." Question to the receiver: "What is this tie you are talking about?" Answer: "Your tie" (tied in a "butterfly"-type bow). The receiver then stated immediately, "And now, about scissors." Question to the receiver: "How did the word 'scissors' come into your mind?" Answer: "I found myself mentally pronouncing the word 'scissors'; it just came to me."

After examining a wealth of such material, the commission concluded that "the perception of mentally transmitted images always enters the subconscious of the percipient [receiver] in the form of hidden . . . [unobserved] processes; a secondary reflected process appears in his consciousness." As a result the image as actually perceived gets more or less distorted.

The commission members concluded also that subconscious processes affect not only what is perceived by the receiver, they also affect the sending process.

More frequently, it was not the actual image ... that was transmitted but images that have some fortuitous association with it. ...
Successful transmission very often does not depend on the
sender's will. ... [One can be] full of eager desire to transmit ...
to the percipient, and this may produce no effect whatever. Con-
versely it frequently happens that details and associated images
are transmitted to which the sender paid no attention while fixat-
ing the object. ... [31]

One of the commission members, R. Desoille, believed there
were four possibilities that might account for how information could be
transmitted from sender to receiver, which is represented in Figure 2.[32]

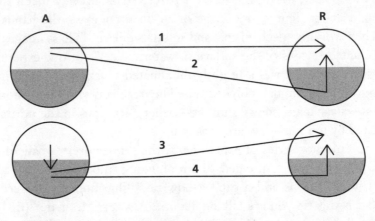

Figure 2

Four possible methods of transmission of thoughts from sender or agent (A)
to receiver (R). The light half of circle represents the conscious mind; the
darkened half represents the unconscious or subconscious mind.

1. Direct transmission from the conscious mind of the sender or
agent (A) to the conscious mind of the receiver (R).

2. Transmission from the conscious mind of A to the subconscious mind of R and then to R's conscious mind.

3. Transmission from the conscious mind of A to his or her own
subconscious mind and then to R's conscious mind.

4. Transmission from the conscious mind of A to his or her subconscious mind, then to the subconscious mind of R, and finally to R's conscious awareness.

Desoille believed it impossible to decide which of these interconnections is occurring in any given case. Vasiliev, who was centrally involved in the commission's work, believed all four types take place, but that "there is a good deal to be said in favor of the fourth alternative," which involves the subconscious mind of both sender and receiver.

Psychologist Christine M. Comstock points out that Freud also believed that communication between people could take place entirely on an unconscious level. "It is a very remarkable thing," Freud wrote, "that the Unc. [sic] of one human being can react upon that of another, without passing through the C's [sic]. This . . . fact is incontestable."[33] Comstock believes unconscious-to-unconscious communication is a basis for exchanges of information at a distance. "This form of communication takes place forcefully and instantaneously," she states, "can happen on the telephone or at other times when the people are not in direct contact."[34] If so, there seems no reason why we cannot pray for others during dreams.

CAN WE *RECEIVE* PRAYERS DURING DREAMS?

Researchers Stanley Krippner and Montague Ullman experimented for a decade with "dream telepathy" at Brooklyn's Maimonides Medical Center. Volunteers spent one or more nights in a sleep laboratory, and were awakened when their brain waves and eye movements indicated they were dreaming. In some experiments they would attempt to dream about a picture postcard that would be randomly selected the following day. Or they would be asked to dream about a picture that had been randomly selected after they had gone to bed and was being focused on by a "sender" in a distant room.

Some of these experiments resulted in impressive correlations. One night *Repast of the Lion*, a painting by Henri Rousseau, was selected as the dream target. In it a lion is biting into the body of a smaller animal. The dreamer had several dreams about violence and animals. In one dream about dogs, "The two of them had been fighting before. You could kind of see their jaws were open and you could see their teeth. . . .

It's almost as though blood could be dripping from their teeth." For this particular dreamer, judges confirmed that five of eight dreams corresponded to the image that was "sent." The odds against a chance explanation was over one thousand to one.[35]

Though not conclusive, these studies strongly suggest that one's unconscious, dreaming state can be a window through which the thoughts of others may enter. If an image on a postcard can "get through," why not prayer?

UNCONSCIOUS PRAYER AND UNREMEMBERED DREAMS

Healing events sometimes suggest that the prayer for healing has originated in the unconscious mind during sleep but is not associated with a remembered dream.

Psychologist Lawrence LeShan, an avid experimenter and authority in distant healing, relates the following incident, which was "the most dramatic single result" in his long experience:

> . . . a man I knew asked me to do a distance [*sic*] healing for an extremely painful condition requiring immediate and intensive surgery. I promised to do the healing that night, and the next morning when he awoke a "miraculous cure" had occurred. The medical specialist was astounded, and offered to send me pre- and post-healing X rays and to sponsor publication in a scientific journal. It would have been the psychic healing case of the century except for one small detail. In the press of overwork, I had forgotten to do the healing! If I had only remembered, it would have been a famous demonstration of what can be accomplished by this method.[36]

In discussing this disconcerting event, LeShan says, "Coincidence has a long long arm and the unexpected *does* often happen." But this may not have been a coincidence. It seems likely that the patient's request for prayer was not dismissed altogether but shoved to the back of LeShan's mind. If so, it could have emerged during sleep to cause LeShan to experience empathic, prayerful concern for the man's situation, which he did not remember on waking—a kind of unremembered dream. This would conform to Desoille's pathway #3 or #4 in Figure 2, in which transmission of mental effects is hypothesized to originate in the unconscious mind of the "sender" before affecting the "receiver."

Although based on suggestive laboratory findings, this is speculation—but so, too, is the "explanation" of coincidence and ascribing the healing to "the natural course of the disease," whatever that may mean. There are other possibilities. Someone else might have been praying for the man's healing, or he might have been praying for himself. Or this may have been a profound example of time-displaced prayer—prayer occurring in the future that is shaping the present—a possibility we shall examine in chapter 7.

Critics may object that the Soviet experiments and the thousands of similar studies done in other laboratories around the world deal with the transmission of "thoughts," not prayers. But thoughts transmitted to others are never "just" thoughts; in many instances the "sender" experiences an empathic, unitive connection with the "receiver" that is similar to the feelings of connectedness commonly experienced in prayer. Thus there seems no reason in principle *not* to extend the implications of the Soviet-type experiments to prayer.

PRAYER WITHOUT CONSENT: ETHICAL ISSUES

Serious questions arise in the wake of the above experiments, which seem clearly to show that mental activity can be used to influence people nonlocally, at a distance, without their knowledge. As we shall see, scores of experiments on prayer show that it also can be used to great effect without the subjects' awareness. The question arises, however, about whether it is ethical to use these techniques if recipients are unaware that they are being employed. This question becomes even more urgent when we see in chapter 9 that prayer can be used at a distance to *harm* people without their knowledge.

Some people, including some scientists, maintain that one should never pray for another without his or her consent; to do so would be a violation of personal rights. Institutional review committees, whose job it is to oversee the design of experiments involving humans and to ensure their safety, have sometimes insisted that the subjects in prayer experiments be told they are being prayed for before the experiment begins.[37]

Should we always obtain consent before praying for another? What does "consent" really mean? Whatever answer people *consciously* give about whether they wish to be prayed for, it is their *un*conscious mind that may have the final say. Psychologist Lawrence LeShan, who has experimented extensively with distant, prayer-based healing, states, "Curiously, belief in the efficacy of healing of this type does not seem to be a factor. Our results seem to be as good with skeptics as they are with believers."[38] In other words, what people believe consciously about the desirability and effectiveness of prayer may not matter. Perhaps deeply held ideas make the vital difference about whether or not prayer or any other distant mental influence is allowed to "get through." While the conscious mind is saying, "Prayer can't work and I reject it. Don't pray for me; I don't want it!" the unconscious may be shouting, "I am in need! I accept any form of healing that works. Please pray for me!"

If it is the unconscious mind that is the subject's gatekeeper, how do we obtain consent from it? Clearly we cannot. Should we then not pray? Surely this would be carrying the principle of consent to the absurd. How then should we proceed?

There are no simple guidelines. Perhaps the Buddhist injunction, "Have good intent," is the best guide. Or the Christian equivalent, the Golden Rule, "Do unto others as you would have them do unto you." We may not always know when or whether prayer is desired. I would maintain that as long as our efforts are filled with compassion, caring, and love, there is little reason to fear that our prayers for others without their consent are somehow unethical.

THE MYSTERY REENCOUNTERED

Penetrating so many secrets, we cease to believe in the unknowable. But there it sits, nevertheless, calmly licking its chops.

—H. L. Mencken[39]

Again we encounter the unknowable—for, try as we might, we can never fully plumb the depths of the unconscious and understand its role in prayer and healing. This *mysterium* is simply inerad-icable; try as we might, we shall not be able to abolish it.

Acknowledging this mystery leads not to a forlorn but to a glori-ous conclusion—for the unknown is the approach to the sacred, the spiritual, the unnameable, the *numinous*. To honor this dimension *is* to be healed. As Jung described, "The approach to the numinous is the real therapy and inasmuch as you attain to the numinous experiences you are released from the curse of pathology. Even the very disease takes on a numinous character."[40]

Chapter 4

Where Do Prayers Go?

God is a sphere whose center is everywhere and whose circumference is nowhere.

—Hermes Trismegistus

One of the most common beliefs about prayer is that it is always "sent" to someone in need, or to the Almighty, who forwards the desired effect. This seems to make sense: We are here; the person in need is there; and the prayer must somehow travel the intervening distance and "get through" to the needy person. Prayer thus resembles radio, television, and telephone signals, all forms of energy that are transmitted across great distances. We embody these images when we make comments such as "I'll be praying for you and sending you energy!"

But there is no evidence whatsoever in any of the experiments on prayer that anything is "sent," or that energy of any kind is involved. If prayer were a conventional form of energy, it should weaken as distance is increased, and this does not happen. If it were energy, its effects could be shielded, but this has not proved possible. This strongly suggests that prayer does not involve any conventional form of energy or signal, that it does not travel from here to there, and that it may not "go" anywhere at all.

If prayer does not go anywhere, then it may simultaneously be present everywhere, enveloping sender, object, and the Almighty all at once. Physicists have a word to describe a world in which information is not sent, but that exists everywhere all at once: *nonlocal*. Although this kind of world may sound like science fiction, a reality of this sort has been proved to exist in modern physics, our most accurate science. These developments rest largely on an idea in physics called Bell's theorem, introduced in 1964 by the Irish physicist John Stewart Bell, and the experiments that have come after it. Bell showed that if distant objects have once been in contact, a change thereafter in one causes an immediate change in the other—no matter how far apart they are, even if they are separated to the opposite ends of the universe. It is important to realize that nonlocality is not just a theoretical idea in physics; it rests on actual experiments.

Some physicists believe that nonlocality applies not just to the domain of electrons and other subatomic particles, but also to "our familiar world of cats and bathtubs," to borrow physicist Nick Herbert's phrase.[1] A growing number of physicists think that nonlocality may even apply to the mind. Again, physicist Herbert, in his *Quantum Reality:* "Bell's theorem *requires* our quantum knowledge to be non-local, instantly linked to everything it has previously touched."[2]

In my book *Recovering the Soul,* I discussed evidence from a wide variety of sources, including everyday experiences, suggesting that consciousness is nonlocal. This picture of the mind is quite different from that given in contemporary biology and medicine, which says that the mind is limited to the brain and to the present, and that it will perish when the body dies. But this cannot be entirely true, for there are simply things that "mind" can do that "brain" cannot. The nonlocal view suggests that the mind cannot be limited to specific points in space (brains or bodies) or in time (the present moment), but is infinite in space and time; thus the mind is omnipresent, eternal, and immortal. If minds are indeed nonlocal, this means that in principle they cannot be walled off and separated from one another: at some level they are unitary and one.[3]

Many people respond jubilantly to this picture of human consciousness. They conclude that if minds are nonlocal and unified, then people can communicate instantly at a distance. Some writers have jumped to the conclusion that physics thus "proves" the existence of prayer, telepathy, and other activities involving communication at a distance, and perhaps permits two-way traffic between human minds and God. But when it comes to nonlocality, the universe has a surprise up its sleeve: in a nonlocal world *it seems to be impossible that a previously thought-out message could be sent from one entity to the other*. In fact, *one can never know ahead of time* what these instantaneously correlated changes between distant entities will be; it is *only in retrospect* that we know they have taken place, by reading a record or measurement of some sort that tells us what happened.[4] Thus physicist Herbert states, "It is difficult to see what use we could make of such non-local connections. On the other hand, *perhaps these connections are not there for us to 'use'*" [emphasis added].[5]

This can seem agonizingly paradoxical, particularly to us Americans, who are famous around the world for our aggressive, rough-and-ready "cowboy" approach to life. This robust attitude invades our thoughts about the nonlocal, unitary connections described by modern physics: What can we *do* with them? What are they *good* for?

If prayer is nonlocal, as it seems overwhelmingly to be, does this mean that it too cannot be "used"? Most people who pray are convinced that prayer *can* be used purposefully; the essence of petitionary and intercessory prayer seems to be the *intentional* use of prayer on behalf of one's self or another. When we pray for a particular outcome—for a cancer to go away, for a heart attack to resolve itself—and it happens, it appears that we *have* used prayer in a purposeful, goal-specific manner.

But prayer does not need to be "used" in specific ways in order to work, and specific messages do not always need to be sent. Open-ended entreaties that employ invocations such as "Thy will be done," "Let it be," or "May the best thing happen in this particular circumstance"— methods we will examine in discussing the Spindrift experiments in chapter 5—do not involve "using" prayer for specific outcomes, nor do they involve sending complicated messages. They are more like an *invitation* for prayer's effects to manifest or show up. Seen from this perspective, perhaps nonspecific prayer strategies do *not* violate physics' prohibition on sending messages nonlocally.

Telesomatic reactions (discussed in chapter 2) demonstrate how we can interact profoundly with each other without sending messages.

They are eerily analogous to the nonlocal events studied by physicists that involve subatomic particles: once these particles have interacted, thereafter a change in one involves an immediate change in the other, regardless of how far apart they may be. Telesomatic events also occur between "entities" who "once interacted" in the past—parents and children, siblings, twins, spouses or lovers—between whom a strong empathic bond exists. The "correlations" that take place between distant people are in the form of shared bodily sensations, thoughts, or actual physical changes. But in all these examples—the mother who experiences a burning sensation when her distant daughter burns her hand in a college chemistry class, or the mother who develops a suffocating feeling when her distant child falls into the swimming pool—neither party is trying to "send" a message or any type of information to the other; they are not trying to "use" their connectedness. Neither do they know at the time that the correlations are happening. It is only later, when they compare their experiences, that they discover for sure that they have occurred. Just as in the physicists' experiments, the correlations are determined only in retrospect; they cannot be engineered in advance. The parallels, then, between what physicists observe in experiments with nonlocality and what humans experience in telesomatic phenomena are extremely close.

The spontaneous, unplanned nature of telesomatic reactions suggests a Law of Reversed Effort, as Aldous Huxley once put it. The more we try to push and control these events, the more they seem to elude us. The secret seems to consist in *not* trying and *not* doing, allowing the world to manifest telesomatically *its* wisdom, not ours.

Is there a lesson in nonlocality and telesomatics for prayer? Could a Law of Reversed Effort exist? Do we connect most profoundly with others in prayer when we cease trying to "make it happen," and might prayer work best when we try least? Perhaps this is what some people mean when they advocate, "Let go and let God." Many people recognize in their own prayer lives a spontaneous, uncontrollable quality in answered prayer—such as a Methodist minister who said, "When I pray, 'accidents' happen." Some authorities not only deemphasize "telling the world what to do," they warn against any degree of self-consciousness whatsoever during prayer. The Benedictine monk Brother David Steindl-Rast captured this effortless, natural approach. "As long as you know you are praying," he said, "you are not praying properly."[6] Trappist monk Father Thomas Keating expresses much the same point. "Silence is the language God speaks," he says, "and everything else is a bad translation."[7] Meister Eckhart's thirteenth-century observation also fits: "Nothing in all creation is so like God as stillness."

Some people don't like this "hands-off" approach to prayer. It seems too passive, too inactive. But if answers to prayer come freely and unbidden when we try least—when we pray in the mode of *silence* of which Father Keating speaks, or when we pray *unconsciously*, as Brother Steindl-Rast implies—this may represent a genuinely *benevolent* feature of the world for which we should be grateful. Rather than complaining that this form of prayer is too passive to suit us, we should give thanks that we do not have to furnish wisdom or foresight to the universe; the requisite information is already present and does not depend on us.

In summary there are close analogies between the nonlocal quantum domain studied by physicists and the "Let it be," "Thy will be done" approaches embodied in many spiritual traditions. Among them:

1. Although correlations occur between distant particles as if they are in intimate contact, physicists cannot purposefully send messages to manipulate their invisible, nonlocal, subatomic world. Similarly, although prayer is effective nonlocally at a distance, we cannot always "make it happen" by willful intent or by praying for specific outcomes.

2. Knowledge that nonlocal correlations have occurred in physics experiments can be determined only in retrospect. Similarly, we usually know that nonlocal events have occurred between humans only after the fact, by comparing experiences once they have taken place.

3. Aggressive activity does not favor the emergence of nonlocal events, either in the physics laboratory or in human experience. Physicists arrange experiments almost as "invitations" for nonlocal events to display themselves. We can also see prayer as an invitation, a respectful request for the world to manifest in benevolent ways.

Chapter 5

How to Pray and What to Pray *For*

Everyone prays in their own language, and there is no
language that God does not understand.

—Duke Ellington

I say, put on your gloves and fight 'em [viruses], go ten
rounds. You have to beat it. . . . You have to challenge
AIDS. . . . I do combat against my virus. Sometimes I go
into my body and I fight my cells and I defeat them. . . .
I didn't get to the leader yet in my dreams, but I know
he'll have . . . every kind of weapon you could think of,
machine guns, bazooka, power pack, everything.
. . . When I kill him, that will cure it in real life.

—Joe Louis Lopez, young person with AIDS

I deal with this disease by looking at it as one of the best
teachers I've ever had. I treat it with respect. I try to love
it. I talk to it. I'll say: "You are safe with me. Do not
worry. I do not hate you." I am not sure if befriending
this virus within me has any healing impact, I know that it
helps me to carry on. If my attitude is good and I am
happy and generous, I feel I can live with this virus within
me for a very long time.

—young person with AIDS

A well-known author and authority on prayer was giv-
ing a seminar. A man in the audience recognized that this was a unique
opportunity that might not come his way again. During the question-
and-answer period, he raised his hand and boldly asked, "Doctor, how
should *I* pray?"

89

"It's very simple," the noted expert responded without hesitation. "Ask God."

This man's question reveals a widespread belief that there is a "best" way to pray. Is there? Even in experimental studies suggesting that prayer is effective, the precise method of praying is almost never controlled or specified. A typical example is cardiologist Randolph Byrd's study in the coronary care unit of San Francisco General Hospital (discussed in chapter 11), in which the various prayer groups were simply told *to* pray, not *how* to pray. Included were Protestants and Catholics, who presumably did not follow the same method. The frequency and duration of the prayers, the nature of the images held in the mind, and the specific goals (if any) of the prayers were left to the preference of each individual.

Perhaps it is understandable that experimenters are reluctant to dictate how one should communicate with the Absolute, and therefore don't give praying subjects specific instructions on how or when to pray. What is more difficult to understand, however, is that the methods that are employed are practically never described in the reports of the experiments, and no tabs are kept on the effectiveness of different methods of prayer.

Imagine that a physician has successfully used penicillin to treat a sick person. A colleague of his has a patient who needs the same treatment. She asks, "What dose of penicillin did you use and how often did you administer it?" The first physician replies, "I really can't say; I didn't record the facts in the patient's chart. Sorry. I guess you're on your own." We would consider this unforgivable, but this is not unlike the situation that results from the failure of most experimenters to document methods of prayer.

PRAYER STRATEGIES:
THE PERSONALITY FACTOR

Pray as you can, not as you can't.
—Dom Chapman[1]

The urge to pray seems so constant and widespread throughout history, it appears to be innate. This suggests that it would be difficult if not impossible to extinguish it. Unfortunately, throughout world history, wars, crusades, and inquisitions have seen to it that we pray in very specific, "correct" ways. As a result there are a great number of prayer dropouts—people for whom the prescribed way just doesn't work.

"Heathen" Meditation and "Aerobic" Prayer: Lessons from Research

Herbert Benson of Harvard University Medical School was one of the first medical researchers to study the health benefits of prayer and meditation. Benson originally studied meditators of the Transcendental Meditation (TM) movement, which was founded in the United States by Maharishi Mahesh Yogi. Working with his fellow researcher, physiologist Robert Keith Wallace, Benson showed that when subjects meditated with a mantra—an Oriental word that contained no meaning for the meditator, but that with use became charged with ritualistic value—healthful bodily changes occurred—lower blood pressure, slower heart rate, and lower metabolic rates.

Benson believed there was no magic in the mantra. To test this suspicion, he taught people to meditate using the word *one* or any other phrase they found comfortable. He then studied Christians and Jews who prayed regularly. He asked Catholics to use as their "mantra" phrases such as "Hail Mary, full of grace" or "Lord Jesus Christ, have mercy upon me." Jews mainly used the peace greeting "Shalom," or "Echad!" meaning "one." Protestants frequently chose the first line of the Lord's Prayer, "Our Father who art in heaven," or "The Lord is my shepherd," the opening of the Twenty-Third Psalm. All of the mantras worked, and all were equally effective in stimulating the healthful physiological changes in the body that Benson called the "relaxation response." But Benson also found that those who used the word *one* or similar simple phrases did not stick with the program, while those who used prayers rather than meaningless phrases continued.

Benson also found a connection between exercise and prayer. He taught runners to meditate as they ran, and found that their bodies became more efficient. Soon there were small groups of runners and walkers using "aerobic prayer," short prayers in cadence with their steps.[2]

Over the years Benson has pursued these findings with theologians, sociologists of religion, born-again psychologists, the Dalai Lama, Billy Graham backers, ecumenicists, and various monastic orders. With a research partner, psychologist Jared Kass, an experienced meditator of the Conservative Jewish tradition, Benson invited thirty priests, ministers, and rabbis to the Mind/Body Medical Institute at Boston's New England Deaconess Hospital. They were presented the scientific evidence that prayer and meditation could change the body in healthful ways, and were taught which forms of prayer elicited this response. On putting this instruction to the test, most of the religious pros got into a "praying high" and became very enthusiastic. One said, "This is why I came into church work in the first place, and I'd lost it."[3]

Benson's research showed not only that prayer is good for the body, but that people's choices of methods of prayer vary widely. His work reveals that prescribing "one right way" to pray can disenfranchise people from the prayer process and result in prayer dropouts.

Benson's work has been elaborated on by others. Psychophysiologist and gifted healer Joan Borysenko, who helped found the Mind/Body program at Harvard, describes several methods of prayer and meditation in her book *Fire in the Soul* that will appeal to a variety of people. [4] Another excellent resource is the book *Full Catastrophe Living* by Dr. Jon Kabat-Zinn, of the University of Massachusetts Medical Center in Worcester.[5]

Questions remain. Why do some people prefer a single prayer word, others a short phrase, and still others elaborate soliloquies? Many theologians, religious scholars, and psychologists have turned their attention to modern psychology in search of answers.

The Psyche's Great Divide:
Introverts and Extroverts

Swiss psychologist Carl Jung further developed the ancient idea that there are fundamental, innate differences in the human personality. He elaborated this theme in his book *Psychological Types*, published in 1920, which was based on twenty years of research. Jung described a watershed in the study of human personality. On one side there are the *extroverts*, who are outer-directed and action-oriented people, and on the other side are the *introverts*, who are more inner-directed and contemplative. Jung found four other major personality differences as well, which he called the four "functions." Two were rational functions—*feeling* and *thinking*. ("Feeling," however, was not to be confused with "emotion," but was more akin to the word *evaluating*.) The other two were irrational or nonrational—*intuition* and *sensation*.[6]

Jung maintained that we are born with one of the four functions dominant and another working in close support of it. Because the other two functions do not feel natural, we push them out of awareness into the unconscious. But that does not mean that they vanish; they continue to exert tension or create inner conflict that may be felt as fear, worry, anger, impatience, or hatred. One of the most common ways of dealing with these rejected qualities is by *projection*—attributing to others our own unacceptable traits rather than acknowledge that they exist in us. Our greatest task, Jung claimed, is to integrate all these different qualities. Only in this way can we eliminate the inner tension and warfare between our conscious and unconscious functions. The price for *not* reconciling them can be immense—unhappy, neurotically conflicted individuals, who when brought together, create a collective conflict that at its extreme results in warfare.[7]

Personality Types: Nature, Nurture, or Both?

A debate has raged for years in the psychology world over whether these traits are present at birth or acculturated. Depth psychologist June Singer states, "Jung seemed to believe that these differences might be present at birth as part of the 'psychological constitution' of the infant, at least in the sense of predispositions toward certain types of attitudes and . . . behaviors "[8] Singer, who has been highly instrumental in the development of Jung's ideas, has provided compelling case histories to support Jung's position. Although it could be shaped to a certain degree by the nurturing effects of parents and environment, she believes the infant's innate predisposition exerts immense influence on the developing personality irrespective of all other factors.[9]

We may think psychological types and personality differences are concerns only of psychologists and "disturbed" people, but we all encounter these differences constantly. Every time we have to relate to a person of a different type, there is tension. Singer says of such an encounter,

> The typical symptom is a cry of exasperation on one side or the other, "I just can't seem to understand you," or "You haven't the slightest idea of what I'm talking about," or, as Mary Magdalene said of Jesus Christ Superstar, "I don't know how to love him." On the international level, nations can spend months deciding on the shape of a table at which they are to sit down to discuss peace negotiations, and then, years later and millions of words later, it appears that they have moved no closer to accord than when the question was whether the table should be round or square. Different types, individually or collectively, operate from different premises.[10]

Parents who do not understand that there can be innate differences in the temperament of children, and who value one temperament over another, may see their child as being somehow wrong, and may try to force the child into a style of behavior to which he or she is not by nature inclined. In this situation, Singer maintains, "a neurosis will almost always occur."

From Personality Types to Spiritual Types

If parents can make children neurotic by failing to honor their innate psychological predispositions, what about those we trust to parent the soul and spirit—our priests, ministers, and rabbis? If they value one way of praying over another; if they exert pressure for everyone to conform to a certain prayer style; if they see nonconformists as misguided or sinful—a "prayer neurosis" can develop. People feel guilty and inadequate, incapable of "true" prayer, estranged, and out of step with their religion: hence prayer dropouts.

The idea that "spiritual types" exist is not new. The Venerable Augustine Baker, a seventeenth-century Benedictine contemplative, knew clearly that different people were predisposed to different methods in approaching the Absolute. In this revealing passage, written almost four centuries before Jung, he seems to be describing extroverts and introverts:

> Those souls who have not a propensity to the interior must abide always in the exercises, in which sensible images are used, and these souls will find the sensible exercises very profitable to themselves and to others, and pleasing to God. But others, who have the propensity to the interior, do not always remain in the exercises of the senses, but after a time these will give place to the exercises of the spirit, which are independent of the senses and the imagination and consist simply in the elevation of the will of the intellective soul to God . . . the human spirit in this way aspiring to a union with the Divine Spirit.[11]

Baker demonstrates here a profound sensitivity to personal differences in attitudes to prayer. He does not recommend that people be what they are not. Although he clearly favors the introverted or "interior" approach that goes beyond "sensible images," those extroverts not inclined this way may follow their own path, in which case they will discover it "very profitable" to themselves and "pleasing to God" as well. Our culture is not so permissive. "In this country our social, educational, industrial, military, and governmental way of life is . . . biased to the . . . extroverted, sensing, thinking, judging types," write Monsignor Chester P. Michael and Marie C. Norrisey in *Prayer and Temperament: Different Prayer Forms for Different Personality Types*.[12] So too are our attitudes about prayer.

As an incurable introvert, I have recoiled all my life at being told by extroverts how to pray. After growing up in a religious tradition that was highly extroverted, I recall the joy I experienced on discovering the contemplative, inner-directed traditions of the East. Concepts such as the Tao—the perfect Way of nature that is indwelling, invisible, and silent—struck a chord long silent in my heart. And the Eastern idea of enlightenment—waking up to what *already* is present—seemed utterly natural and true. These concepts seemed to require not action or doing but *understanding*—something that held immense appeal to me. I later discovered in the writings of Evelyn Underhill and others that these were not just Oriental ideas, as Westerners often believe.[13] For centuries there has been a similar mystical, contemplative, inner-directed tradition in Christianity, whose essential tenets can hardly be distinguished from those of the East. As only a single example, Buddhist scholars have suggested that the ideas of Meister Eckhart, Germany's great mystic of the thirteenth century, bear the closest resemblance to the key ideas in Buddhism and Taoism.

Shyness and Prayer

There may be a genetic basis for introversion and extroversion. Ongoing research by psychologist Jerome Kagan of Harvard University suggests that some people may be predisposed toward shyness from birth. He and his colleagues have studied the behavior of more than 350 infants over the past twelve years. They suggest that in shy infants there is a low threshold for stimulation of a part of the brain's limbic system, called the amygdala, which helps regulate emotional responses. This means that stressful stimuli result in a more marked physical impact. When shy, inhibited infants confront even mildly stressful events, they display exaggerated activity of the sympathetic nervous system, such as large increases in heart rate and dilation of pupils. In contrast outgoing infants are "low-reactive"—they do not demonstrate such marked physical responses to stress. Although these researchers propose that biological differences may predispose children at a very early age to introversion or extroversion, they are quick to point out that biology is not destiny, and that other factors are involved. Early environmental factors, such as the love and caring of parents, are also undeniably powerful factors in shaping personality.[14]

Introverts and Extroverts:
Pilgrims on the Same Path

Jung believed that the healthiest personality was one in which the various factors had been acknowledged and integrated into a functional whole. Thus if one surveys the history of the great religions, one finds many contemplative mystics who have become action-oriented achievers as well. Examples include St. Teresa of Avila, Julian of Norwich, and St. Hildegard of Bingen. These inner-directed figures shook

Christendom to its foundations with their words and actions because they were not *just* introverts, but individuals who harmoniously integrated *both* the introverted and extroverted aspects of their personality.

It may seem, nonetheless, that I have advocated the introverted approach to prayer excessively in these pages. Perhaps this is unavoidable; I write about the territory I know best. Yet I cannot overemphasize that introversion and extroversion are not pure states, but simply predispositions. Were this not so, communication would be impossible and conflicts would be unresolvable.

"LET IT BE" OR "MAKE IT HAPPEN"?
THE SPINDRIFT STUDIES

The Spindrift organization in Salem, Oregon, has for a decade performed simple laboratory experiments showing that prayer works.[15] After proving that prayer is effective, they proceeded to investigate which type of prayer strategy works best. One of their most important contributions is the distinction they make between *directed* and *nondirected* prayer. Practitioners of directed prayer have a specific goal, image, or outcome in mind. They are "directing" the system, attempting to steer it in a precise direction. They may be praying for the cancer to be cured, the heart attack to resolve itself, or the pain to go away. Nondirected prayer, in contrast, is an open-ended approach in which no specific outcome is held in the mind. In nondirected prayer the practitioner does not attempt to "tell the universe what to do."

Which prayer technique—directed or nondirected—is more effective? It is important always to bear in mind that *the most important discovery of the Spindrift tests is that prayer works and that both methods are effective*. But in these tests the *non*directed technique appeared quantitatively more effective, frequently yielding results that were twice as great, or more, when compared to the directed approach.

This may surprise people who favor the techniques of directed imagery and visualization that are quite popular today. Various authorities on imagery contend that if the cancer or heart attack is to be cured, a specific image must be employed as to how the end result will actually come about. Some studies have suggested that the more robust and aggressive the image is, the better the outcome. But Spindrift's tests suggest that the situation is more complex.

Spindrift devised an experiment to put directed and nondirected prayer to the test. The study involved growing a mold on the surface of the kind of rice agar plate bacteriologists and mycologists routinely use. The mold was stressed by washing it in an alcohol rinse so as to damage it and retard its growth, but not enough to kill it. A string was then placed across the mold, marking it into sides A (the control side) and B (the treated or prayed-for side). When directed prayer was used to encourage the growth of side B, nothing happened; growth remained static. But when directed prayer was replaced by nondirected prayer, in which no goal was held in the mind of the healer, side B began to multiply and formed additional concentric growth rings.

As a result of numerous tests on a variety of biological systems, the Spindrift researchers suggest that healers will be most effective if they strive to be completely free of visualizations, associations, or specific goals. Physical, emotional, and personality characteristics should be excluded from thought, they say, and replaced by a "pure and holy qualitative consciousness of whoever or whatever the patient may be."[16] It is this method that they refer to as genuine spiritual healing. Methods that rely on directed prayer, in contrast, are referred to as "psychic" healing, "faith" healing, "mental" healing, or the placebo effect—all of which, they claim, depend on suggestions to the patient that he or she will improve.

An obvious question arises concerning nondirected prayer: If one does not pray for a specific result, how can one tell if the prayer is answered? Spindrift believes, on the basis of a large number of tests, that when a nondirected prayer is answered, the outcome is always in the direction of "what's best for the organism."

This was demonstrated in a series of germination experiments in which the practitioner did not know what was best for the seeds involved. One batch was oversoaked and thus heavier than it should have been for proper germination to occur; another batch was undersoaked and lighter than optimal. The seeds were being evaluated early in the germination process according to changes in weight (properly germinating seeds gain weight early in germination). Ideally the oversoaked seeds should have eliminated excess water early and become lighter, and the undersoaked seeds should have absorbed water and become heavier. Not knowing which batch was which, the practitioner could not "tell the seeds what to do," so he used nondirected prayer and trusted that the seeds would simply move toward the norm according to what was best for each seed. The nondirected approach worked. The results showed that the oversoaked beans eliminated water and lost weight, and the undersoaked beans gained water and increased their weight. On the basis of this type of experiment, Spindrift believes that an *answered* nondirected prayer is one in which the organism moves toward those states of form and function that are healthiest for it.[17]

I am uncertain about generalizing these conclusions to human beings. What is "best for the individual" may sometimes involve death, not life, as in the case of someone with a horribly painful condition that is clearly beyond cure, and for which all pain medication has ceased to work. In such a situation, I believe that a nondirected prayer for that person could be answered by demise.

It is not easy to employ a nondirected prayer strategy. When our health fails, we usually waste no time in telling the universe what to do. We want the cancer to vanish, the pain to subside, the high blood pressure to resolve. Even if we *try* to follow a nondirected approach, we may have a hidden agenda: "I'll pray nondirectedly, but I wouldn't *mind* a cure!"

This is the way in which, as scholars Ann and Barry Ulanov describe in their book on prayer, *Primary Speech*, "God becomes a big jukebox prayer wheel and our prayers the coins that operate the machine." But the "jukebox prayer wheel" does not always play our selection: "Prayers are sometimes answered by the experience of more struggle, by our being plunged into situations where we must risk more than we ever dared before."[18]

The Spindrift experiments have important implications for those situations in which we simply do not know what to pray for. Suppose we want to control our physiology in a way that promotes healing of a particular problem. Should we image or pray for an increase or decrease of blood flow to a specific organ? For an increase or decrease in a specific type of blood cell? For a rise or fall in the blood concentration of a particular chemical? These questions can be bewildering to specialists, let alone laypeople. The Spindrift experiments are consoling on this point. They suggest that it isn't always necessary to know how the body ought to behave for healing to occur. One need only pray for "what's best"—the "Thy will be done" approach.

In discussing these findings in lectures and seminars, I find that many people who have favored the *directed* approach to prayer and visualization often jump to hasty conclusions on hearing the Spindrift experiments. They say to themselves, "I must be praying wrong. I should switch to the nondirected approach." This misses the point. Spindrift's most important contribution is showing that prayer works, not that everyone should suddenly start praying, imaging, and visualizing identically.

There may have been subtle factors in the Spindrift experiments, such as the personality of the praying people, that were not examined. After becoming personally acquainted with some of the Spindrift experimenters, my feeling is that, by and large, they are wonderfully introverted. Thus it appears to me quite reasonable that the nondirected prayer method worked best, because this felt most natural and authentic to them. If these experiments were repeated using extroverts instead of introverts, perhaps the *directed* way of praying would have proved superior. Thus the very worst use we could make of these studies would be to say, "Science has now shown that there is 'one best way' to pray." The most important lessons are that prayer works and that *there is no formula*, no "one best way" to pray that everyone should follow.

NONDIRECTED PRAYER: THE IMPORTANCE OF SURRENDER

Janet Quinn, R.N., Ph.D., of the University of Colorado School of Nursing, is a leading nurse theorist, educator, and researcher in the field of noncontact Therapeutic Touch. She has deep experience in working with very sick people of all sorts, including people with AIDS. Dr. Quinn has discovered the value of *surrender* in these patients, which is an important element in the nondirected approach we've been examining. She observes that, when patients first come to see her, they

> very much [want] to be in control and [take] charge.... [But AIDS] is utterly unpredictable.... There are lots of ways to respond.... One way is to get completely hopeless and give up.

And the other is to surrender. . . . Surrendering is incredibly empowering because it is an action. And giving up is the refusal to take action. Giving up is saying there is nothing else to do. . . . To surrender is absolutely active and requires doing over and over again. Surrender is not something that's done once and for all. You can't say, "I surrender to AIDS today . . . or I surrender to God." It's required minute to minute. Being surrendered is becoming extraordinarily active in one's process. . . . Surrender increases the quality of life . . . and the quality of one's dying. There is a peacefulness that comes with that . . . versus the despair that comes with giving up.[19]

Even though nondirected prayer strategies employ no specific goal, they are not to be equated with a completely blank state of mind, totally free of all images, visualizations, attitudes, or thoughts. Certain Buddhist schools, for example, advocate "clear mind" as a goal in meditation, yet they employ techniques that are rich in mental imagery. In one mind-clearing exercise, we are asked to imagine that we are sitting quietly by a stream. When a thought enters our awareness, imagine that it is a floating log, just coming into view upstream. Observe the log floating nearer, without becoming attached or involved with it in any way, and finally let it float away and out of sight downstream. The goal in this technique is not to fight the images or try to banish them entirely, but simply not to be pushed around and dominated by them.

Just so, nondirected prayer does not require us to wipe the slate of the mind totally clean. We may still experience feelings, emotions, and images, but not as specific goals or preferred outcomes.

UNIVERSAL TECHNIQUES IN PRAYER AND IMAGERY

For direct influence of remote systems, the most effective form of intentionality appears to be one that is goal-oriented and thorough, yet not excessively effortful or egocentric. Excessive striving seems to produce additional distractions or noise that interferes with goal-accomplishment. The effectiveness of this form of

> intentionality points to the reality of a truly teleonomic,
> goal-directed process in Nature that complements the
> more familiar process-oriented, causal principles.
>
> —William G. Braud[20]

Some of the most remarkable laboratory experiments showing the ability of people consciously to change the world around them are the human interconnectedness research studies at the Mind Science Foundation in San Antonio, Texas. We examined some of these studies in chapter 2, and saw that individuals could bring about significant changes in certain physical functions in distant people, with whom sensory contact was impossible.

How do they do it? What mental techniques do they use? On close inspection these strategies can't be called *either* directed *or* nondirected. In addition to whether or not goals and preferred outcomes are held in the mind, other factors seem to be involved. Dr. William G. Braud of Mind Science Foundation lists five simple but powerful techniques that expand considerably the concepts of directedness versus nondirectedness in prayer and have direct application to the way we pray: relaxation and quietude, attention training, imagery and visualization, intentionality, and strong positive emotions. Braud notes that these techniques are frequently used by mystics, who have incorporated them for centuries in their methods of praying.[21]

Relaxation and Quietude

In virtually all their experiments, the Mind Science researchers begin by asking the participant simply to relax. There are many methods of doing this—stress-management books are filled with them. Relaxation is a skill that can be cultivated with practice. It is not simply a feeling that stays in the mind; it ushers in a host of body-wide physical changes that indicate a state of low physiological arousal.

Attention Training

Paying attention to any object—whether an actual physical thing or the object of one's prayer, imagery, or visualization—

sounds simple, but it is quite difficult to sustain for any length of time. As anyone who has tried to do so quickly realizes, the mind tends to wander wildly—likened by St. Teresa of Avila to riding a bucking horse. But with practice one can acquire the skill of sustained and focused attention. When this occurs a sense of oneness and unity frequently develops between the person who is praying, imaging, or visualizing, and the object or person to whom these efforts are directed.

People who achieve success in laboratory experiments utilizing imagery, visualization, or prayer frequently describe a feeling of actually bonding with the object they are trying to influence, whether a machine, animal, or human. Some of the earliest subjects in biofeedback experiments at Harvard Medical School were frequently asked how they managed to control bodily processes that ordinarily operate silently and invisibly—blood pressure, heart rate, skin temperature, and so on. They were unable to verbalize how they did it. But when the researchers asked them how they *felt* when they did it, they began to make statements that sounded genuinely mystical—"becoming one" with the biofeedback instruments that were measuring the bodily processes, "fusing" with the entire surroundings, and so on.

In Braud's analysis, focused attention does more than create pleasant feelings of oneness and unity. "Focusing attention upon any object," he states, "establishes a two-way communication channel with that object—a channel that can be used to gain knowledge about that object or to influence it."[22] After one has opened the channel, images provide the vehicles for carrying information back and forth through that channel.

Imagery and Visualization

What is imagery? Psychophysiologist Jeanne Achterberg has given one of the best definitions: thinking without words.[23] "Imagery" is often used synonymously with "visualization," but there are differences. Researcher and clinician Patricia Norris of the Voluntary Controls Laboratory of the Menninger Clinic in Topeka, Kansas, states that although both involve "wordless pictures" in the mind, visualization is used to imply deliberately constructed wordless thoughts directed toward a desired goal.[24]

As we have seen, the Spindrift experiments ignited a healthy debate over whether goal-free or goal-directed visualizations work best in prayer. Again, rather than enshrining one method over the other, the most important realization is that *both* work. It is important to choose the method that intuitively *feels* best. Highly specific, goal-directed prayers seem unnatural, even arrogant, to many people who may feel it isn't proper to "tell God what to do." Other individuals prefer an aggressive, robust, "make it happen" approach that involves highly specific and goal-directed prayers and visualizations. As we have already seen, personality factors are undoubtedly involved in these preferences, such as the levels of introversion and extroversion present in one's psyche. These personality traits are extremely resistant to change and tend to be stable across a lifetime. We should acknowledge them for what they are, and take them into account in our personal prayer strategy.

Intentionality and Strong Positive Emotions

Western cultures have valued one form of intentionality above all others: a robust, aggressive, "go for it" style of *making* something happen. Even at play we are told to be decisive and effortful. But other cultures, particularly those of the Orient, have for millennia recognized an effortless way of effecting change in the world—a "doing without doing" in which one cooperates with the natural order instead of trying to change it. This way of being allows "controlled accidents" to happen magically—the archer's arrow hits the mark, the artist achieves aesthetic perfection, and so on. This approach recognizes an intrinsic order in the world that may manifest if we attune or align with it in a certain way.

Our form of intention is important, but so too is the level of emotion. Simply put, feeling strongly about something helps us accomplish it. "Strong," however, does not mean an outwardly showy demonstration of feeling. Strong emotions may be felt quietly and inwardly. Like the great surges of current in the ocean's depths, they need not disturb the surface.

THE POWER OF A *DIRECTED* APPROACH IN PRAYER

If we left our examination of prayer methods at this point, our analysis would be incomplete. Everyone has heard of dramatic examples of healing in which highly specific, *directed* strategies were used in imagery and prayer. In one well-known example, the person imaged her cancer as a piece of red meat, and her immune cells as a pack of ravenous wolves who attacked the meat and destroyed it. Another successful imagery motif involved visualizing cancer cells as helpless, frightened fish and the immune cells as voracious sharks feeding on them.

Although stories such as these are anecdotes and do not count as hard evidence, we would be foolish to ignore them. In their support there is ample solid scientific evidence that directed, highly specific imagery can bring about changes in the body. For instance, Dr. Howard Hall of Pennsylvania State University has shown that subjects, using hypnosis, can generate a more active immune response when they imagine their white blood cells as "strong and powerful sharks."[25] Working with 126 cancer patients, psychophysiologist Jeanne Achterberg and psychologist G. Frank Lawlis demonstrated that the patients' clinical response—future tumor growth or remission—was directly related to the specificity, vividness, strength, and clarity of their mental imagery. The work of Achterberg and Lawlis, pioneers in the clinical use of imagery, thus offers another side to the debate over whether directed or nondirected imagery and prayer strategies work best.[26]

In several additional studies, subjects have been able to affect the behavior of some immune cells and not others, when mentally imaging the activity of these different cells in highly specific ways. For example, Drs. Achterberg and Mark S. Rider examined the ability of subjects to affect specifically the numbers of certain types of white cells—neutrophils and lymphocytes—in the bloodstream. (Neutrophils and lymphocytes make up about 85 percent to 90 percent of the total white-cell count in the blood.) Thirty subjects were randomly assigned to either the "neutrophil" or "lymphocyte" group, and underwent a six-week

training program during which they focused on images of the shape, lo-
cation, and patterns of movement of these cell types. Music was used to
enhance their imagery. Counts of various types of white blood cells
were made before and after their final twenty-minute imagery session.
Results showed that the neutrophils (but not the lymphocytes) decreased significantly in the neutrophil group, while the lymphocytes
(but not the neutrophils) decreased significantly in the lymphocyte
group. The authors concluded that the highly directed imagery was
cell-specific; that is, it affected the cells toward which it was intended or
directed, and not others.[27]

Dr. G. Richard Smith and his colleagues at the University of
Arkansas College of Medicine reported what is perhaps the first fully
documented case of a human being intentionally changing the immune
system. It involved a thirty-nine-year-old woman who was able to
change her positive skin test for varicella zoster (the chicken pox virus)
at will—from positive toward negative, and then toward positive, a feat
she repeated six months later. She used a rather specific form of imagery,
imagining the redness and swelling surrounding the skin test getting
smaller and smaller, while sending "healing energy" to the area.[28]

The experimental support for the effectiveness of mental imagery
in general as well as for directed, specific imagery is too voluminous to
cover here. Comprehensive reviews of this material are now available
from many sources. Particularly valuable are the internationally known
works of Achterberg and Lawlis, mentioned above, and Anees A.
Sheikh, professor and chairman of the Department of Psychology at
Marquette University and past president of the American Association
for the Study of Mental Imagery.[29]

PRAYER: SOUND OR SILENCE?

Why is prayer so noisy?

—Anne N., age three

The belief in the power of words is universal and is
embodied in creation myths worldwide. "In the beginning was the
word," we say in the West. According to an ancient Egyptian creation
story, the Creator's first act was to pluck a reed, slit its tip, and write the

world into existence. The Australian aborigines describe how the Creator first emerged from the formless void and sang the world into existence—words put to music. These myths relate Word and World—and thus many traditions have maintained that, if we are to know God, we must ourselves become involved with words, with the language of God.

Yet there has always been a competing point of view that has emphasized the value not of words but of silence. This perspective sees words as obstructions to deeper connections with the Universal. Chuang Tzu, who helped craft the tenets of Taoism in ancient China over two millennia ago, suggested that the most profound forms of communication go beyond words. In his typically provocative way, he said, "Words exist because of meaning; once you've got the meaning, you can forget the words. Where can I find a man who has forgotten words so I can have a word with him?"[30]

How would we moderns possibly know whether there is any value in wordless silence? Quietude in our age is in short supply. We seem to *need* noise. This fact was vividly demonstrated to me when my physician colleagues and I were designing a new medical office. We were discussing whether or not we should have music piped through the waiting room and other public areas. We could not agree, and eventually invited a salesman of built-in sound systems to discuss with us the advantages. The salesman could tell we were dubious. Drawing himself up with total confidence, he made his final pitch, the argument that would sweep away all our objections. "Gentlemen," he solemnly proclaimed, "you do not realize that *the worst thing in the world is silence!*"

Because we have so little tolerance for quiet, silence and prayer seem incompatible to many people, and wordless prayer is a contradiction in terms. It was not always so. The anonymous author of *The Cloud of Unknowing* did not specifically urge wordless prayer, but nonetheless recommended brevity:

A man or woman, suddenly frightened by fire, or death, or what you will, is suddenly in his extremity of spirit, driven hastily and by necessity to cry or pray for help. And how does he do it? Not, surely, with a spate of words; not even in a single word of two syllables! Why? He thinks it wastes too much time to declare his urgent need and his agitation. So he bursts out in his terror with one little word, and that of a single syllable: "Fire!" it may be, or "Help!"

Just as this little word stirs and pierces the ears of the hearers more quickly, so too does a little word of one syllable, when it is not merely spoken or thought, but expresses also the intention in the depth of our spirit. . . . And it pierces the ears of Almighty God more quickly than any long psalm churned out unthinkingly. That is why it is written, "Short prayer penetrates heaven."[31]

When we are confronted with anguish, pain, or illness—when we feel as if we *must* pray—we are not likely to deliberate about whether or not we shall pursue a specific or nonspecific approach, or whether sound or silence is more appropriate. In the immediacy of the moment, we simply *pray.* As psychobiologist Joan Borysenko states in her incisive book *Guilt Is the Teacher, Love Is the Lesson,*

When we are absolutely miserable, prayer is no longer a dry rote repetition. It becomes a living and vibrant cry for help. It becomes authentic. In pain we forget the "thee's" and "thou's" that keep us separated from God, and reach a new state of intimacy that comes from talking to God in our own way, saying what's in our heart.[32]

Chapter 6

Love and Healing

> The main reason for healing is love.
>
> —Paracelsus (1493–1541)

If scientists suddenly discovered a drug that was as powerful as love in creating health, it would be heralded as a medical breakthrough and marketed overnight—especcially if it had as few side effects and was as inexpensive as love. Love is intimately related with health. This is not sentimental exaggeration. One survey of ten thousand men with heart disease found a 50 percent reduction in frequency of chest pain (angina) in men who perceived their wives as supportive and loving.[1]

The power of love to change bodies is legendary, built into folklore, common sense, and everyday experience. Love moves the flesh, it pushes matter around—as the blushing and palpitations experienced by lovers attest. Throughout history "tender, loving care" has uniformly been recognized as a valuable element in healing.

David McClelland, Ph.D., of Harvard Medical School, has demonstrated the power of love to make the body healthier through what he calls the "Mother Teresa effect." He showed a group of Harvard students a documentary of Mother Teresa ministering lovingly to the sick, and measured the levels of immunoglobulin A (IgA) in their saliva before and after seeing the film. (IgA is an antibody active against viral infections such as colds.) IgA levels rose significantly in the students, even in many of those who considered Mother Teresa "too religious" or a fake. In order to achieve this effect in another way, McClelland later discarded the film and asked his graduate students simply to think about two things: past moments when they felt deeply loved and cared for by someone else, and a time when they loved another person. In his own experience, McClelland had been able to abort colds with this technique. As a result of his personal experiences and research, he became an advocate for the role of love in modern healing.[2] He once told a group of his medical colleagues,

> I can dream a little about changing hospital environments, one that relaxes you, gives you loving care, and relieves you of the incessant desire to control and run everything. A healthful environment. Certain doctors, nurses, social workers—all of us—can learn ... that being loving to people is really good for their health. And probably good for yours too.[3]

But can love and caring do more than act *within* a person? Is it powerful enough to act at a distance *between* individuals, overcoming separation in space and possibly in time? Can love unite people over geographical distances even when the "receiver" is unaware that love is being offered? This is a way of asking if prayer works; because when one person prays for the welfare of another, the person who prays is extending compassion, empathy, and love. Can these qualities genuinely "reach out"?

One of the greatest scholars and researchers in the history of parapsychology, F. W. H. Myers, was struck by the fact that people who were "telepathic" with each other—people who could share thoughts at great distances—were frequently connected emotionally with one another deeply and lovingly. Myers concluded that love, empathy, and compassion somehow made it possible for the mind to transcend the limitations of the body. Love was so important in this process that Myers honored it by giving it a place in a natural "law." As he put it,

"Love is a kind of exalted but unspecialized telepathy; —the simplest and most universal expression of that mutual gravitation or kinship of spirits which is the foundation of the telepathic law."[4]

Virtually all psychic healers who use prayer agree. They claim uniformly that distance is not a factor in the healing power of prayer, and most of them state emphatically that love is the power that makes it possible for them to reach out to heal at a distance. During attempts at healing, healers generally feel infused by love and transformed by caring. This feeling is so pronounced that they typically describe "becoming one" with the person being prayed for. In his landmark study of psychic healing, *The Medium, The Mystic, and the Physicist*, psychologist Lawrence LeShan—who is perhaps the greatest living authority on the subject—reported the observations of several famous healers:

> In Agnes Sanford's words, "Only love can generate the healing fire." Ambrose and Olga Worrall have said, "We must care. We must care for others deeply and urgently, wholly and immediately; our minds, our spirits must reach out to them." Stewart Grayson, a serious healer from the First Church of Religious Science, said, "If this understanding is just mental it is empty and sterile" and "the feeling is the fuel behind the healing." Sanford wrote: "When we pray in accordance with the law of love, we pray in accordance with the will of God."[5]

In addition to the beliefs of healers that love is vital if prayer is to "get through" and facilitate healing, considerable evidence, both laboratory-based and anecdotal, suggests that empathy somehow connects distant organisms. These entities are of a vastly different variety, ranging from microorganisms to human beings. This fact is important. If empathy indeed connects a vast range of living things, it may be a built-in feature of the natural world, not just a human quirk or perhaps an erroneous observation.

EMPATHIC CONNECTIONS

Empathy, compassion, and love seem to form a literal bond—a resonance or "glue"—between living things. The following observations suggest that when empathic connections are present, feelings experienced by one entity may be felt also by another, in spite of considerable spatial separation.

J. B. Rhine and Sara Feather, of the Parapsychology Laboratory at Duke University, collected fifty-four "returning animal" cases. Some of them are quite astonishing because there is no obvious way the animal could have known the way back home. Thus these are not "homing" events, as demonstrated by pigeons. An example is the case of Bobbie, a young female collie. She was traveling with her family from Ohio to Oregon, the site of their new home. Although the family had made the trip previously, Bobbie had not. During a stop in Indiana, Bobbie wandered, became lost, and could not be found. Finally giving up the search, the family proceeded. Almost three months later, Bobbie appeared at the doorstep of the new home in Oregon. She was not a "lookalike" dog; she still had her name on her collar in addition to several identifying marks and scars.[6]

In another case a young boy named Hugh Brady, who kept homing pigeons as pets, found a wounded pigeon in the garden of his home and befriended him. He nursed the bird back to health and gave him an identification tag marked #167. The next winter Hugh suddenly became ill, was rushed to a hospital two hundred miles away, and underwent surgery. While he was still recovering, on a bitterly cold, snowy night he heard a tapping at the window. Hugh summoned a nurse and asked her to open it. In flew a pigeon, which landed with a flutter on Hugh's chest. He identified his bird immediately by sight, which was confirmed by the tag number. Pigeons are well known, of course, for their homing ability; but #167 was not homing. He was traveling to a place he had never been.[7]

Not only does empathy influence relationships between living things, it is apparently involved in human-machine interactions. In a series of experiments extending over the past decade, researchers at the Princeton Engineering Anomalies Research (PEAR) Laboratory at Princeton University have studied the ability of people to influence the behavior of random physical events occurring in different mechanical devices, such as a microelectronic random event generator (REG). This device produces a string of binary samples, or bits, at a rate of one thousand per second, in trials of two hundred bits each, and counts the number that conform to a regular positive or negative alternation. A human operator sits in front of this device and views on a display the sequence of numbers, and tries to influence the output distribution in either a positive or negative direction—in other words, trying to will the machine's output up or down. In addition to the REG, many other mechanical devices are employed in the PEAR Lab experiments.[8] Over the years fifteen pairs of individuals have been tested in 256,000 attempts to influence the REG. Their results have been compared to those of ninety-one individual operators, who have generated 2,520,000 trials on the same device. The results indicate overwhelmingly that both individuals and couples working in concert can influence the REG, steering its output from sheer randomness toward a particular pattern. The most successful pairs are couples who are deeply attached emotionally and empathically to each other—so-called "bonded" couples.

This database, the largest of its kind ever collected, is impressive evidence that empathy and emotional closeness allow the emergence of a power that is capable of shaping physical events "out there" in the world. This is supportive evidence for the claims of the prayer healers above: "Love [empathy, compassion, caring, bonding] is the fuel behind the healing."

In the Princeton studies, empathic effects are not confined to bonded couples. Individual operators also describe an emotional bonding with the machines they are trying to influence. Some say they "become one" with the device while they are trying to influence it.

The PEAR experiments show clearly that *the effects of empathic bonding transcend space*. It simply does not matter whether the operator is sitting in front of the instrument in the same room at Princeton University, or whether he or she is on the other side of the world or somewhere in between (these experiments have actually been carried out at global distances). The subject is equally effective, regardless of spatial separation from the device.

These studies show also that *the effects of empathic bonding transcend time*. In a remarkable variation of these experiments, the PEAR experimenters ask the operators to influence the output of the REG device *before* it has actually run. The results are the same as if they are sitting before the device, trying to influence its behavior while it is running in real-time. They also ask the operator to influence the machine's output *after* it has run. That is, the machine will run and the subject will try to influence its output at some *later* time. Results are identical to efforts made in the present. This is shocking—an example of cause *following* effect—because we presume that past events are fixed and cannot be influenced.

The PEAR experiments do not stand alone. They are supported by similar experimental findings by physicist Helmut Schmidt, which show that subjects can influence the output of a microelectronic random event generator *after* the machine has run (see chapter 7).

Does empathy help prayer "get through"? "Getting through" presumes that there is such a thing as a separate person fundamentally isolated and distinct from every other. This concept may be flawed. As the eminent researcher in parapsychology Stanley Krippner has stated,

> Another posture could be taken . . . ; namely, that *all* consciousness is basically "group consciousness." An individual's awareness, attention, memory, etc., is socially constructed. Without group interaction, an individual would never achieve "identification" with anyone or anything. From this viewpoint, "group consciousness" is the fundamental matrix from which "individual consciousness" emerges.[9]

We have for so long defined ourselves as separate personalities that we have fallen into the hypnotic spell of believing that separation, not unity, is the underlying reality. But if *unity, not separation, is fundamental*, then at some level of the psyche *nothing* may be "getting through" because there are no separate parts for something to get through *to*.

If this is so, the connections we feel with others during prayer are "nothing special." We do not have to establish or invent these connections because they already exist. Prayer is not an innovation, it is a process of remembering who we really are and how we are related. From this point of view, there is good reason to rid prayer of its aura that it is some rare state we enter only on certain occasions. If the unity it connotes is not the exception but the rule, there should be no celestial halo surrounding prayer.

This also implies that at certain levels of the psyche, there is no such thing as "distant" healing because there is no distance separating people that must be overcome. This means that healing of another is in some sense self-healing, for the spatial distinctions between "self" and "other" are not fundamental. Perhaps that is why it always feels good to love another, and why our prayers for others are also good for us.

LOVE'S PARADOXES

Man can try to name love, showering upon it all the names at his command, and still he will involve himself in endless self-deceptions. If he possesses a grain of wisdom, he will lay down his arms and name the unknown by the more unknown . . . by the name of God.

—C. G. Jung[10]

Of all the trivialized concepts in this so-called New Age, perhaps the greatest involves love. Books pour from the pens of well-meaning patients and doctors alike, attesting to its phenomenal power in healing. Love melts away tumors, cures addictions, banishes fear, catalyzes miracles, transform lives—all this we are told *ad infinitum*. If we could only learn to love and forgive ourselves and others and let go of all our fears, grudges, and hatreds, our health would be better. Paracelsus's dictum, "The main reason for healing is love," frequently becomes distorted into "The *only* reason for healing is love." The frenzied enthusiasm surrounding love has led to one of the greatest ironies of the New Age, namely, that significant numbers of sick people are made to feel guilty in the name of love for not being well.

About ten years ago, a patient of mine developed a breast lump and had a mammogram and breast biopsy, which revealed cancer. Considerably shaken, she sought help from a psychological counselor well known for dealing with newly diagnosed cancer patients. This man was deeply convinced that all physical ailments reflected emotional and spiritual shortcomings. On my patient's first visit, the counselor, without bothering to inquire deeply about her history and psychological makeup, stated abruptly, "There are only three possibilities for why you have cancer. You either don't *love* yourself enough, you have some deep seated *fear* you're not in touch with, or you are not *trusting* enough of yourself and others!" Deeply introspective, my patient felt the counselor's observations were simply wrong. "Having cancer is difficult enough without the guilt trip," she said. She rejected his analysis and found help elsewhere. Ten years later, after using orthodox cancer therapy as well as continued inner psychological work, she has no trace of illness.

This is not to suggest that I do not believe in the role of love in healing. As I have explained, I believe it is vastly important, particularly in prayer-based healing. I only want to point out that love should not be enshrined as some magical, monolithic principle in health and healing. When it is, the sick person often pays.

At some point one wants to stand up and demand of all the love merchants, what do you *mean* by love? There is a tendency in holistic health circles to regard it simply as an emotion that has something to do with unconditional caring, compassion, and empathy. This is fine as far as it goes, but it is only a partial picture. The ancient Greeks, for example, believed that love was the domain of Eros—and Eros was, above all, mysterious and paradoxical. As Jung explained, "In classical times, when such things were properly understood, Eros was considered a god whose divinity transcended our human limits, and who therefore could neither be comprehended nor represented in any way." [11] In contrast to most New Agers, the Greeks recognized that many of Eros's qualities were decidedly not nice. Jung agreed. As a result of observing the actions of Eros in the lives and dreams of thousands of his patients, he concluded that Eros was a "daimon, whose range of activity extends from the endless spaces of the heavens to the dark abysses of hell . . . [and which contains] . . . incalculable paradoxes. . . . "[12]

A lot of New Age literature has stripped love of its complexity and sanitized it into something nice that can be made into a simplified formula everybody can understand. Love's mysterious, darker qualities are relegated to the shadows or completely ignored.

The Old Testament story of Job is about the shadow side of love, and how one can be victimized by a loving God. Job's story should be required reading for those who today insist on linking spiritual perfection and health, for it shows that horrible things can happen to blameless people, and that the currently popular love formulas for health are sadly incomplete.

We are told at the outset that Job was "perfect and upright" (Job 1:1). In other words he did nothing to deserve his fate. But in spite of Job's perfection, God allowed terrible things to be done to him—his ten children were killed, his wealth destroyed, his health replaced by a disfiguring, painful disease. If we believe that "God is love," then we are forced to conclude that love must be an extremely complex phenomenon—Jung's "daimon" in action.

Things haven't changed much since Job's time: people who are highly spiritual, God-realized, and "enlightened" still become ill. In order to "keep God's skirts clean," as Alan Watts once put it, we hear various rationales for these troubling events. Some say that the sick person only *appears* loving, trusting, and free of fear, but deep down, real problems exist that he or she isn't "in touch" with. Or that the sick are living out their karma and "paying back" for transgressions in past lives, or that they "chose" this illness in a previous life, and so on. One gets the feeling that these are desperate, ad hoc attempts to preserve the love-model of health rather than confront the obvious: the model is flawed; love is no guarantee of health, longevity, or anything else but paradox and deep mystery.

What do we really *know* about the place of love in healing? What can we say without undue fear of contradiction? We can demonstrate experimentally that love, compassion, caring, and empathy catalyze healing events, and that this power operates at a distance and outside of time. But we know also that love is compatible *with* illness—in the same sense in which Jesus said, "Love your enemies," not "Don't have any."

Love occupies a majestic place in healing. Lying outside space and time, it is a living tissue of reality, a bond that unites us all.

Chapter 7

Time-Displaced Prayer:
When Prayers Are Answered
Before They Are Made

And it shall come to pass, that before they call, I will
answer.

Isaiah 65:24

But what is now? There is no such thing in physics. . . .
No physical experiment has ever been performed to detect the passage of time. The most profound puzzle of all
is the fact that, whatever we may experience mentally,
time does not pass, nor does there exist a past, present,
and future. . . . the notion of a moving time makes virtually no sense . . . in spite of the fact that it dominates our
language, thoughts, and actions.

—Paul Davies, *Other Worlds* and *Space*
and Time in the Modern Universe

Our concepts of prayer follow the precepts of classical,
Newtonian physics, in which mind and consciousness play no role.
Events are always guided by the blind, neutral laws of nature, and cause
always precedes effect in the linear, flowing river of time.

Of all the ways "new physics" differs from this classical view, none
is stranger than how subatomic events are conceived to take place.
Consider a radioactive particle A, contained in a box that is shielded

from our view. We know from past experiments that A will give off either particle B or particle C after one minute has passed. We wait the requisite minute, then ask: Which particle was given off? B or C? According to the most widely accepted interpretation of quantum physics, the situation never resolves itself until we actually *look* inside the box in some way. Until then there is only a "superposition" of possibilities, B *and* C. If there is no physical instrument such as a Geiger counter to do the "looking" or recording—or, some say, if there is no human being to examine the recording—the final event never comes to completion, even though we might wait forever for it to do so. Before looking we can only talk about possibilities, not actualities. It is the act of observation, it is said, that brings all the potential happenings into a single result that can be called an actual event.

For several decades researchers have wondered whether reality, if it is tied to the actions of human observers, may to some extent be flexible, susceptible to being shaped by mental effort. Physicist Helmut Schmidt of the Mind Science Foundation in San Antonio, Texas, devised some of the earliest and most precise experiments in which subjects tried to influence the output of random event generators (REGs), devices that operate on the basis of truly random radioactive decay or electronic noise, such as occurs in semiconductors. These devices can be made to express their randomness by strings of ones and zeros that are converted into lights or sounds, which the subject tries to influence. This is an indirect way of influencing what nature is doing at the subatomic level.

Schmidt's studies, done over many years, suggest strongly that humans can mentally influence the behavior or output of random event generators. How good is Schmidt's data? Esteemed statistical psychologist Hans Eysenk and Cambridge researcher Carl Sargent estimate that the likelihood against Schmidt's results being due to mere chance are several million to one.[1] Even skeptics have been impressed. Ray Hyman, a well-known critic of parapsychology, has said of Schmidt's work,

> By almost any standard, Schmidt's work is the most challenging ever to confront critics such as myself. His approach makes many of the earlier criticisms of parapsychology research obsolete. [I am] convinced that he was sincere, honest, and dedicated to being

as scientific as possible . . . the most sophisticated parapsychologist that I have encountered. If there are flaws in his work, they are not the more obvious or common ones.[2]

Schmidt's work has been replicated independently by other researchers. Researchers Dean Radin and Roger D. Nelson analyzed the results of over eight hundred studies involving random event generators, conducted between 1959 and 1987. Published in the prestigious journal *Foundations of Physics*, their findings indicated unequivocal evidence for a reliable, replicable direct mental influence on these random natural events. They further showed that the effect remained even with increasing refinement of the experiments, and that the results could not be explained away by the "file drawer" effect, in which researchers report only positive experiments and disregard neutral or negative ones.[3]

In a stunning series of experiments, physicist Schmidt found evidence that these influences may be displaced in time. His subjects tried to influence the output of an REG *in the past*—that is, they tried to affect random events that had already been prerecorded but not yet consciously observed. The outcome: "Apparently, present mental 'efforts' were able to influence past events about which 'Nature had not yet made up her mind.'"[4]

Schmidt's experiments appear to indicate that past subatomic events are malleable, capable of being influenced mentally, even though they have already occurred and been recorded in some way, *so long as they have not been consciously observed*. In a fascinating twist to some of his REG experiments, a third party observes the prerecorded subatomic events during the interval between their initial generation/recording and the session in which the mental influence is attempted. Results suggest that such preobservation, if sufficiently intensive, may prevent or obstruct direct mental influence on past events. The ability of observation to "fix the past" has been tested in cases when not only humans, but dogs and goldfish were the observers![5]

CAN WE AFFECT OUR "MEDICAL PAST"?

The most convincing experimental evidence that one can affect the past is in the subatomic dimension, the domain of the

random event experiments of Schmidt and others. This may suggest
that time-displaced effects operate *only* at invisible, remote levels, and
have nothing to do with the large-scale world of human bodies and
organ systems. But in recent years, the physics lab and medical science
have drawn closer together. We now realize that many diseases begin
with disturbances at the subatomic level. For example, melanoma, a
skin cancer, can develop when excessive ultraviolet irradiation triggers a
mutation in atoms in the skin. Abnormal "channels" in various tissues
cause impaired flow of calcium and other ionized particles and lead to
heart disease, hypertension, and other problems. While illnesses thus
may *appear* to begin in whole organs, such as the lungs, heart, or kidneys, their most fundamental site of origin is in the subatomic dimension.

This perspective offers a possibility hitherto unimagined in medicine: 1. if we can affect the dynamic qualities of subatomic particles
through our observations, as physicists maintain; 2. if these efforts can
reach into the past and change unobserved events presumed already to
have happened but about which "nature has not yet made up its mind,"
as has apparently been demonstrated in the above experiments; and 3. if
the behavior of subatomic particles is associated with disease causation,
which we know to be true; then 4. *we may be able mentally to shape our
"medical past" in order to bring about health not illness.*

Science fiction? Psychologist William G. Braud of the Mind Science Foundation studied the ability of one subject to "reach back into
the past" and exert time-displaced influences over his prerecorded electrodermal response, the ability of the skin to conduct an electrical impulse. Although the experiment did not reveal statistically significant
results, intriguing events were noted. When the subject was reminded
that he had, in fact, succeeded in time-displaced experiments in another
laboratory (which he had forgotten), his scoring improved dramatically;
and it dropped precipitously when at one point he intentionally tried to
do *worse* on the task.[6]

If the mind could engage in time displacement, this would raise
serious implications for modern health care. Consider the customary
annual physical exam. Periodic exams intuitively make sense because
they uncover problems before they manifest. Many of us know someone who has had a cancerous lump that was discovered on an annual

exam and was excised before it had a chance to spread; or whose diabetes was discovered in its early stages before it ravaged the kidneys, heart, and blood vessels. But in spite of the fact that annual physical exams make good sense and are recommended by almost all doctors, there is little statistical evidence that they increase longevity in the population as a whole. If they are so dramatically useful in individual cases, why should it be so difficult to prove their benefit across the board?

The annual physical exam and the extensive battery of laboratory tests that goes with it are the quintessential "acts of observation" in modern medicine. In quantum physics, as we've seen, observing and looking convert possibilities and potentialities into actual events and *fix* them irrevocably. Could the same process be happening in the physical examination? Although the cancerous lump is sometimes detected and removed early, could the beneficial result of such an event be swamped by other more serious disease processes that are "locked in place" and fixed by the processes of observation and looking that are part of the annual exam? If so this might explain why it is so difficult to demonstrate the overall effectiveness of the annual health examination.

I recall a case that most physicians will find familiar from their own experience. A poor, uneducated woman came to the emergency room with an obvious breast cancer in an advanced stage. It was ulcerated, as large as a grapefruit, infected, and had spread to the lymph nodes in her armpit, neck, and elsewhere. "How long has this been present?" I asked. "Fifteen years," the poor woman said. I was shocked. I knew from the statistics that one does not live fifteen years after a breast cancer has become visible, if it goes untreated. She was resolute, however, and her family affirmed her claim. "Why have you not seen a doctor to have this treated?" "Because if I did," she said, "the doctor would cut it. This would let air touch the cancer, which makes it 'run wild,' and I would die." Her presentiment proved true. The woman had surgery and died shortly thereafter.

Why was she able to live fifteen years from the cancer's first appearance with no treatment whatsoever? Many modern therapies are not nearly as effective. She seemed to be saying that as long as nothing formal was done, her fate was not fixed. As long as things remained shrouded with unknowns, she had a chance; but looking, observing, and doing would create a downhill, fatal course.

There are several possible explanations for this woman's course. Her denial of cancer may have been a factor that actually favored survival, as in the cases of metastatic breast cancer we examined in chapter 3. Her own fears about surgery may have created a self-fulfilling prophecy leading to death. But in addition, could there be an analogy to the time-displaced effects demonstrated by physicist Schmidt, in which subjects were able to change the past as it unfolded, prior to the observation of the recorded events? The answer may appear to be no, because the woman's cancer *was* observed by her. But the fact is that we do not always know what causes death in cancer. Some people live normal, healthy lives with obvious cancers, and some cancers go away on their own. With cancer, we physicians say, anything can happen as a part of "the natural course of the disease." Perhaps the critical aspects of these processes are *not* observable, not lodged in the cancerous mass itself, but rooted in the invisible subatomic events that ultimately underlie all physiological processes. As long as these events are left undisturbed and unobserved, perhaps the person has more of a chance to control them intentionally in a healthy way, delaying their progress or perhaps neutralizing them altogether.

We may regard the attitude of the woman with breast cancer as unenlightened and superstitious. But warnings about laboratory testing by distinguished leaders in the profession have surfaced for more than a half-century. By the 1940s Tinsley Harrison, the legendary diagnostician and editor of an acclaimed textbook of medicine, called attention to "the present-day tendency towards a five-minute history followed by a five-day barrage of special tests in the hope that the diagnostic rabbit may suddenly emerge from the laboratory hat."[7] Although Harrison was not referring to the effects of observation we are examining, but the departure from patient-centered medical care, his warning may be more appropriate than he realized. And what would he say today, when a patient is sometimes given *less* than five minutes to tell her story, and testing may continue for considerably longer than five days?

Today's Americans are the most medically tested population that has ever lived. No one has ever been probed, x-rayed, biopsied, scoped, and scanned as we. Is there a dark side to these presumed benefits? Can a test actually serve as a "blocking agent" to the beneficent effects of consciousness on the past? Does "medical looking" in all its forms erase the malleability of critical physiological events thought already to have happened? This might help explain why the people of many other nations, who are "examined" far less than we, enjoy a higher level of health and greater longevity.

Let me be clear: I am not arguing against annual examinations and tests. I have seen too many lives saved to suggest that they be abandoned. I have personally had periodic checkups—including tests—for years, and intend to continue this habit. But I believe there may be more here than meets the eye, perhaps more than *should* meet the eye, until after certain precautions have been taken, which I have added over the years to my interactions with my personal physician.

How might these precautions work? Consider, for example, a woman who discovers a breast lump. The doctor affirms it on an examination and advises a course of action that eventually includes a mammogram and a biopsy. Before the tests, *no one knows* what the "real" situation is; only possibilities exist.

At this pre-test stage, if we were to take seriously the possibility that we may be able to reach back into the past and affect the unfolding of subatomic events that precede illness, an interesting scenario might unfold. The patient might take advantage of this window of opportunity and initiate her own prayers, images, and visualizations. She might marshal her friends to do the same—all in an attempt to affect the critical processes in her body *before* a cancer might actually develop. Only after a thorough attempt was made would the process of testing, looking, observing, and interpreting—*fixing* the event—be allowed to proceed.

Another option would be to do nothing—no exam, no tests, no looking and observing of any sort. This was the choice of the woman described above who outlived the statistics for breast cancer. Today a lot of people would do the same, feeling that medical testing is always wrong. I disagree. The fact is that many people, for whatever reason, *cannot* change their medical past and insure benign outcomes. That is why medical testing can save lives.

We could apply these precautions before *any* form of "medical looking"—whether physical examinations, X rays, mammograms, electrocardiograms, exercise stress tests, sonograms, scans of various sorts, and so on. Implementing these interventions need not complicate or delay medical evaluations; in all nonurgent situations, these precautions could be taken before the patient even goes to the physician's office or hospital.

This may seem fanciful; but the evidence suggests, as we've seen, that it *is* possible to reach back into the past and affect the elaboration of subatomic events before they are consciously observed, thus affecting events as they later come to be. I would suggest that this is at least worth the attempt, *especially* since no harm would be done in the process.

A NEW KIND OF PREVENTIVE MEDICINE?

Prayer, imagery, and other types of mental effort that seek retroactively to change small-scale events add a new dimension to the concept of "preventive medicine." Ordinarily, if we want to prevent something from happening, we perform an act in the *present* in the hope of affecting the *future* in a particular way. The above possibilities suggest another side to prevention—trying to shape our "medical present" by intervening in subatomic processes in the *past*, before they have become irrevocably fixed by the process of observation.

Are some people already performing these kinds of actions, perhaps unconsciously? Such a person might be difficult for health professionals to deal with. The patient would continually be interfering with the doctor's "observations," skewing tests and evaluations of various sorts toward a benign result. The test that the physician predicted to be abnormal would turn up normal, and his predictions for a dire outcome would not prove true. These patients would appear cantankerous, always appearing to throw monkey wrenches into diagnostic workups and treatment plans. The fact that the patient's clinical course was excellent would prove baffling to doctors, who could not figure out why the individual always seemed to beat the odds.

All doctors know such people. Jeanne Achterberg describes one of her patients who fits this profile:

[She has] survived five "healthy" years with lung cancer. She drives everyone crazy because she's not doing it right. She's in "denial," she has no social support except therapy groups, she won't go back to work, she has no insight (they say), no reason to live (that anyone can identify with), punitive parents who still beat up on her emotionally, etc. etc. And, she has no imagery that I can figure out, is too anxious to relax or meditate, eats terribly. She's proud of herself, she decides her own medical treatment, wouldn't let them remove her lung. . . . She comes in to see me every week. She teaches me things, and keeps me from getting too arrogant about my advanced knowledge. I love her.[8]

CAN PRAYERS BE ANSWERED BEFORE THEY ARE MADE?

We are, all of us, creatures of parts, used to beginnings, middles, and ends because our lives are divided that way, and our language . . . follows the same logic. . . . But the spirit is one and undivided, without parts, not chained to beginnings or middles or ends, and thus not dependent upon sequential reasoning. . . . Its province, its every-thing, is wholeness.[9]

—Ann and Barry Ulanov, *Primary Speech*

Our beliefs about prayer, as we've noted, always embody a particular "worldview," a set of guiding beliefs about how the universe works. In the United States, our worldview is shaped by traditional, classical physics as described in the seventeenth century by Sir Isaac Newton. One of the primary facets of the Newtonian vision is that time flows, much like a river, in a single direction. This view implies that once something has happened, it cannot be redone; that one can't "go back" in time; and that causes *always* precede effects. Prayers, which are lodged in linear time, must therefore be offered *before* they can be answered.

But as far back as the time of the writing of the Old Testament, time has behaved in strange ways:

Then spake Joshua to the Lord in the day when the Lord delivered up the Amorites before the children of Israel. . . . Sun, stand

thou still . . . ; and thou, Moon. . . . And the sun stood still, and
the moon stayed, until the people had avenged themselves upon
their enemies. . . . So the sun stood still in the midst of heaven,
and hasted not to go down about a whole day. And there was no
day like that before it or after it. . . .

(Joshua 10:12–14, KJV)

In addition to standing still, could time become "disjointed," such
that the future would precede the present, or the present precede the
past? Theoretical physicist John Archibald Wheeler of the Institute of
Theoretical Physics in Austin, Texas, thinks so. He has created what he
calls a "delayed-choice experiment":

[In it] the observer creates not only present attributes of quantum
entities [such as electrons], but also attributes that such entities possessed far back in the past, which by conventional thinking existed
long before the experiment was conceived, let alone carried out.[10]

Physicist Nick Herbert, in his important book *Quantum Reality*,
says,

Wheeler's delayed-choice experiment seems to show that the past
is not fixed but alters according to present decisions. [This ac-
cords with] certain Eastern philosophies [that] have come to a
similar conclusion concerning the creative power of the present
tense: "The moment of the world's creation is seen to lie, not in
some unthinkably remote past, but in the eternal now."[11]

The possibility that time does not always flow in one direction
may have profound implications for our understanding of how prayer is
answered. Consider the following case:

A man diagnosed as having cancer of the colon asked his minister
to pray for his recovery. He was not a religious person and never
prayed for himself. He also was a very private person and had told
no one about his diagnosis, which precluded prayer from friends
and family. When he returned to his physician later the same
week, follow-up studies showed complete disappearance of the
cancer. He wrote a letter of thanks to his minister. When the

dates of the diagnosis, the initial prayer request, the minister's prayer, and the disappearance of the cancer were compared, it was apparent that the cancer had disappeared before the minister had actually prayed for the man. It was unlikely that anyone else prayed for him, since no one knew his diagnosis except him and his doctor, who also was not a religious person and did not pray.

There is no proof in this example, skeptics would say, that prayer had an effect; the cancer could have disappeared "on its own" as part of "the natural course of the disease," or the diagnosis may have been wrong in the first place. But if we make two assumptions—1. that prayer works, for which we will offer considerable evidence later on; and 2. that time may not be one-way—this case may represent an example of *time-displaced prayer*, prayer that is answered before it is made.

In the movie *Terminator 2*, a global nuclear war has wiped out a considerable part of the world's population. This holocaust was caused by runaway computers that took things into their own hands and could not be stopped. In order to "prevent" this cataclysm—which had already happened—survivors of the event went backward in time. They successfully thwarted the computer designers, reshaped the past, and thus created a new future, which did not include nuclear war.

Time-displaced prayer may work like this. Benevolent, compassionate thoughts may reach back into the past and reshape or prevent events such as a heart attack or a painful, protracted illness. As C. S. Lewis put it, "Shocking as it may sound, I conclude that we can at noon become part causes of an event occurring at ten A.M."[12] If this sounds like science fiction, we should realize that the possibility is permitted *in principle* in modern physics, as we've seen.

TIME-DISPLACED ILLNESS

Every stick has two ends.

—Ancient proverb

The case of the patient with colon cancer described earlier illustrates how *good* things seem to happen outside of one-way time. If good things violate the linear time sequence, however, we should be alert to the possibility that *bad* things may do the same.

One of the most difficult things about being a physician is that we are sometimes unable to determine the cause of an illness, in spite of our most fervent attempts. Diseases whose causes are unknown are called "idiopathic." This word comes from the Greek *idiopatheia*, "a feeling for oneself alone," or a suffering for oneself. Because one does not know the cause of an idiopathic illness, it seems to come out of the blue and thus seems random, unfair, unreasonable, undeserved. That is why idiopathic diseases evoke "a feeling for oneself alone." The Old Testament story of Job is our archetypal example of idiopathic illness. Job's lonely, agonizing quest was to find a cause for his suffering, when apparently there was none.

Idiopathic illnesses may appear so unexpectedly and their cause may be so obscure that they seem to erupt from nowhere. They appear to be *an effect without a cause*. This gives them the unique quality of appearing outside the temporal flow. They resemble time-displaced prayer in this regard, but with a difference: rather than having *good* things precede their cause, as in time-displaced prayer, with idiopathic illnesses *bad* or *pathological* events precede their cause.

Examples in which the disease appears to come first and the cause later are exceedingly common in medical practice. For example, Peter was a twenty-eight-year-old artist who went to his physician complaining of a chronic cough. He did not smoke, nor did he have any other risky health habits. His past medical history was perfectly normal. Although Peter's physical exam proved unremarkable, his chest X ray showed changes typical of tuberculosis. Although his doctor felt confident that the diagnosis *had* to be TB, extensive laboratory tests failed to prove the diagnosis. All cultures and microscopic examinations of his sputum for the tuberculosis bacterium were negative, and a skin test for the disease also was normal. Unable to prove TB, the physician embarked on an elaborate diagnostic workup for related possibilities. The results were uniformly normal.

Because Peter's only symptom was a chronic cough, the physician decided simply to follow him closely without treatment for a few weeks. The cough continued, and the doctor decided eventually to repeat the studies. This time Peter's TB skin test was highly positive, and all his sputum cultures grew the tuberculosis organism. Treatment was begun and he recovered completely.

Did Peter's disease precede its cause? Was his a case of time-displaced illness? Because there is no place for time-displaced events in the Newtonian worldview that guides medical science, it is always easier to say that the physician simply missed the diagnosis the first time around; the cause was there but went undetected. Perhaps. Physicians *can* miss diagnoses; lab tests *can* be wrong. But more subtle processes may be at work, processes rooted in the nonabsoluteness of time.[13]

TIME-DISPLACED HEALTH: WHEN GOOD THINGS HAPPEN TO BAD PEOPLE

While Job's experience shows us that good people can experience uncaused *bad* events, there is an extremely common flip side to this scenario: "bad" people can experience a continuous stream of apparently uncaused and undeserved *fortunate* events.

In medical practice good things seem to happen to bad people all the time. All physicians encounter "health reprobates," people who violate every rule of good health but who never get sick. They may smoke three packs of cigarettes a day, drink copious alcohol, follow an atrocious diet, engage in risky behaviors of all types, and live to be a "healthy hundred." Health reprobates challenge all of our ideas of cause-and-effect. For them smoking does *not* lead to lung cancer, emphysema, or heart disease; imbibing massive quantities of alcohol does *not* cause cirrhosis; a high-fat diet is *not* associated with atherosclerosis; reckless sexual behavior does *not* result in AIDS or any other sexually transmitted diseases. Our "explanations" of these situations are superficial. We may shake our heads and say they are "just lucky," or that "their luck will run out one day." There is also the "right genes" hypothesis: they are blessed from birth, protected by a robust constitution that simply "runs in the family."

There are other possible explanations. Any time we see apparent violations of cause-and-effect, we should suspect that a time-displaced event may be occurring. Like the colon cancer that "just went away" without apparent cause when the minister prayed *later* for the patient, similar events might be happening in the futures of health reprobates that continually reshape their present *before* illness can result from their destructive behavior. This would be an interesting form of preventive medicine, in which high-risk candidates for lung cancer, emphysema, and heart disease avoid developing these problems as a result of the influence of the future on the present.

There may be important spiritual lessons here. Because prayer can violate the categories of past, present, and future, it seems timeless. Thus one of its functions may be to awaken us to the "eternal now," the experience of timelessness described by the mystics of every esoteric religious tradition. Perhaps this is one of the lessons inherent in one of the most universal of prayers, "Thy will *be* done." Divisions in time are absent from this prayer: It does not say, "Thy will be done today or tomorrow." "Be" implies the infinitude in time that always has been ascribed to the Almighty. "Thy will be done" denotes an eternal pervasiveness of the Divine will. Perhaps the prayer "Thy will be done" can awaken us to a new way of judging time and a new way of thinking about the role of prayer in health.

Chapter 8

Your Doctor's Beliefs and Why They Matter

> A doctor is not merely a dispenser and synthesizer of sci-
> entific knowledge, nor is a patient an inert receptacle. As
> Norman Cousins said, "Ultimately it is the physician's re-
> spect for the human soul that determines the worth of
> his science."
>
> —Paul Roud, *Making Miracles*

In 1955 a West German physician reported a strange series of events in three of his patients for whom he could do nothing more using standard, orthodox medicine.

One had chronic inflammation of the gall bladder with stones. The second had failed to recuperate from a major abdominal operation and was practically a skeleton, and the third was dying of widespread cancer. The physician first permitted a prominent local faith healer to try to cure them by absent treatment without the patients' knowledge. Nothing happened. Then he told the patients about the faith healer, built up their expectations over several days, and finally assured them that he would be treating them from a distance at a certain time the next day. This was a time in which he was sure the healer did NOT work. At the suggested time all three patients improved quickly and dramatically. The second was permanently cured. The other two were not, but showed striking temporary responses. The cancer patient, who was severely anemic and whose tissues had become waterlogged, promptly excreted all the accumulated fluid, recovered from her anemia, and regained sufficient strength to go home and resume her household duties. She remained virtually symptom-free until her death. The gall bladder patient lost her symptoms, went home, and had no recurrence for several years.[1]

Why did the three patients improve? Based on our observations so far in this book, we can give several possibilities that may have acted alone or in combination:

• The placebo effect—the power of suggestion in the patients themselves—may have been at work.

• The faith healer's initial action may have had a real but delayed effect.

• The faith healer may have continued to exert his activities, even though the physician thought he had not.

• The belief of the physician may somehow have brought about the improvements.

Let's focus on the last possibility. Because it is generally agreed that a patient's attitudes are crucial to his or her response to a particular treatment, it is usually only the *patient's* beliefs that are considered when a particular therapy is entered. Is he or she cooperative? Will he or she give the medication a chance to work? Does he or she have a desire to get better? A will to live? Although it is essential to ask these questions, the beliefs of the patient are only one side of the coin. The physician's beliefs also shape the outcome of therapy, so it is also vital to examine them in any treatment situation.

It is widely known that physicians can fool themselves when they try to determine why patients get better. They may attribute the patient's response solely to the administered drug, when the improvement has actually resulted from suggestion. In order to eliminate this confusion, elaborate experimental methods have been developed, the most common of which is the famous double blind.

In a double-blind situation, experimental subjects don't know which group they belong to, whether to the experimental group being given the active drug, or to the control group being given a placebo.

Neither does the experimenter know which group is which, or who is receiving what. This means that *both* experimenter and subjects are "blinded"—hence double blind. An experiment in which only one of these blinds is employed is a single blind, and a study in which neither is used is a nonblind experiment.

One of the results of these sorts of studies has been the discovery of the power of placebos to bring about dramatic improvements in an astounding variety of conditions—due, it is always said, to the patient's *belief* that he or she is ingesting a powerful substance. But any healing transaction involves at least *two* sets of beliefs: the patient's *and* the physician's.

What about the effect of the doctor's beliefs?

Physicians can exert powerful effects through their beliefs. For instance, if they strongly favor a therapy, they can "talk up" its effects to the patient. This enthusiastic cheerleading can inflate patients' expectations and set the stage for dramatic placebo-type responses, even though the therapy itself may be inherently ineffective. This can be a problem in scientific medical research. In single-blind studies, in which the patients do not know whether they are taking the active medication or a placebo pill, the doctor can unconsciously show more interest and enthusiasm in the "treatment" group than the control group. This can lead, through suggestion, to a heightened response on the part of the treatment group, all due to the doctor's *belief* that they should do better.

So far this is not surprising; the effects of suggestion are well known. But evidence also suggests that a physician's beliefs can alter the results of *double-blind* studies as well, experiments in which he or she does not know which group is which.

Researcher Jerry Solfvin examined extensively the power of the physician's underlying beliefs. In three double-blind studies of the use of vitamin E in treating angina pectoris, the pain associated with coronary artery disease, an enthusiastic doctor who *believed* in vitamin E found it significantly more effective than a placebo,[2] while two studies conducted by *skeptics* showed no effect.[3]

Consider also the facts surrounding meprobamate, one of the earliest minor tranquilizing drugs, marketed in the United States as Miltown and Equanil. During the 1950s there were conflicting reports of its effectiveness. Enthusiasts consistently found that it worked, while skeptics could find no effects beyond those of a placebo. To clarify this situation, researchers designed a double-blind study in which one of the physicians had a "skeptical, experimental" attitude toward the drug, while the other had an "enthusiastic, therapeutic" attitude toward it. They were totally unaware which pills were which, meprobamate or placebo. The patients also were in the dark; they did not even know they were involved in an experiment. The results: meprobamate proved significantly more powerful than the placebo—but only for the physician who *believed* in it. There was no drug effect for the skeptical physician's patients.[4]

This study was repeated, conducted simultaneously at three metropolitan psychiatric outpatient clinics. The results were replicated in two of the three clinics. Overall, therefore, three of the four meprobamate studies suggested strongly that the effectiveness of the drug over the placebo was correlated with the physician's attitudes and beliefs toward it, and that the beliefs of the prescribing physician can somehow penetrate the double-blind conditions of the experiment and shape the action of the drug.[5] Thus Solfvin concludes,

> [S]tudies with a wide variety of treatments have conclusively affirmed that the administering physician or researcher is not independent of the results in double-blind treatment effectiveness studies. . . . *As a general rule, the double-blind cannot any longer be assumed to guarantee the exclusion of the nonspecific effects of the treatment, especially when the actual treatment has a weak or variable effect.* [Emphasis in the original.][6]

This does not mean, of course, that drugs and other therapies cannot work "on their own." The effects of some therapies are so strong that they drown all other factors, including beliefs. If an individual is injected with a thousand units of quick-acting insulin, no matter who believes what, the chances are overwhelming that he or she will become unconscious as the blood sugar plummets. Or if a person ingests food tainted with botulinum toxin, one of the deadliest substances known, death is virtually guaranteed.

Double-blind tests are not useless. They have been and remain a valuable aid in testing therapies of all sorts. But they are not perfect, and these limitations should be acknowledged. *The greatest value of dou-*

ble blinds may lie, however, in their limitations, which reveal something marvelous about us—that there is some aspect of the human psyche capable of shaping events in our world.

WHY DO DRUGS WORK?

If a doctor's beliefs can actually influence the action of medications, as these double-blind studies indicate, how is it possible that a particular drug can have a single, generally consistent pattern of action? Why shouldn't it have two patterns of effectiveness—a positive one for enthusiasts and a negative one for skeptics? Drugs do have general patterns of activity. Penicillin usually works when doctors prescribe it appropriately. Why doesn't the prescribing physician's belief affect its effectiveness?

I can think of at least two reasons. As we've noted, the power of some agents is so strong it can overwhelm all other factors, including beliefs and expectations. Penicillin falls into this category when, for instance, it is used appropriately for streptococcal throat infections. The second reason that drugs may work consistently is that, over time, physicians' beliefs about them become consistent. A consensus develops and a community of enthusiasts forms, shaping what the drug will do, as in the double-blind experiments above.

For centuries physicians have recognized that new drugs can seem highly effective when first introduced, but stop working after a while. This phenomenon led the famous nineteenth-century French physician Armand Trousseau to observe, "One should use a new drug as often as possible, while it still has the power to heal."

We can imagine a possible scenario consistent with the double-blind experiments above, whereby the effectiveness of a new medication would be reduced. Typically new drugs are marketed with sensation, hype, and fanfare, whipping up enthusiasm among physicians and shaping its effects positively. But when other factors begin to enter the picture, including the beliefs and expectations of patient populations as well as the information about the drug's side effects, negative reports begin to circulate. The community of physician-enthusiasts are thus converted toward a more skeptical stance. As beliefs about the medication swing toward the negative, the drug's effectiveness diminishes.

MEDICINE IN DENIAL

Let something appeal to us and we will make sense out
of it. Let something offend us, disturb us, threaten us and
we'll see that it doesn't make sense.
—Jule Eisenbud[7]

If such an effect is real it would throw doubt on all empirical findings since Galileo.
—Martin Gardner[8]

Doctors and scientists in general react with horror to
the possibility of such "experimenter effects," a reaction reflected in the
quotation by Martin Gardner above. The possibility that a physician's
thoughts and beliefs could actually shape a patient's physiological responses—at a distance, even when the patient is unaware—is unthinkable. This has resulted in a virtual blindness in modern medicine to
these issues, and an unconscious drive to deny demonstrated facts.

It is not hard to imagine why. It is much more comfortable psychologically for a physician *not* to have to consider the effects of his or
her thoughts and beliefs on what is occurring. All the emphasis can remain on expertise and technique. Moreover a physician who honors the
evidence that his or her beliefs *can* shape a patient's physical responses
has in effect acknowledged the existence of a genuinely nonlocal, Era
III–type event (see chapter 2). This means admitting that while the
brain acts locally, consciousness can act at a distance. And this calls into
question some of the bedrock assumptions of the physician's training
and his or her views of how the world works.

In 1949 psychologist Donald O. Hebb enunciated a position that
still dominates neuroscience:

Modern psychology takes completely for granted that behavior
and neural function are perfectly correlated. There is no separate
soul or lifeforce to stick a finger into the brain now and then and
make neural cells do what they would not do otherwise. . . . One
cannot logically be a determinist in physics and biology, and a
mystic in psychology.[9]

Although written almost a half-century ago, Hebb's view that consciousness is inseparable from the functioning of individual brains remains the cornerstone of physiological psychology.[10] Materialistic positions such as these abound; they are part of the credo of modern medicine. There is no room in them for physicians' beliefs to affect nonlocally the outcome of therapy.

These points of view are usually ingrained at deep emotional levels. They reflect one's worldview, self-concepts, and basic attitudes about consciousness. These are high stakes. Rather than modify or dismember these deeply held beliefs, it is frequently easier to dismiss or deny the validity of anything that challenges them. This is not surprising. Scientists and physicians, like the rest of us, have an emotional need to believe they are right, free of bias, and open to evidence of any kind.[11]

CHOOSING A DOCTOR

The beliefs of the patient and the doctor ideally should coincide. The *best* possible situation is one in which both parties genuinely and honestly believe a therapy is going to be effective. The *worst* is one in which there is a collision or conflict between the two sets of beliefs, or in which neither the physician nor patient feels that the therapy is going to work. In the latter case, two sets of negative beliefs are shaping the outcome of therapy, which can set the stage for therapeutic disaster.

Acknowledging the power of belief to shape outcomes in therapy should encourage doctors to examine critically their behavior toward patients. Many physicians cultivate an attitude of remoteness, aloofness, and noninvolvement with their patients. Some appear morose, even chronically depressed, as if expecting the worst. Doctors usually defend these behaviors by referring to "the burdens of the profession," or by claiming that one can do one's best only by remaining emotionally detached. It is also common for doctors to paint the worst possible outcome. If things turn out better than predicted, the physician is a hero and the patient is grateful. This is known in the profession as "hanging crepe"—*black* crepe, as if at a funeral. This does not always involve deception; many doctors *are* pessimists and naturally expect the

worst. The custom of giving the "cold facts" to patients following diagnosis, grimly detailing one's statistical chances of survival with cancer,
heart disease, AIDS, and so on, is also common. Many physicians believe they are actually presenting a positive picture when they recite
"survival data." But patients who hear such comments as, "You have a
25 percent chance of surviving this cancer" frequently interpret them
to mean, "I have a 75 percent chance of dying."

If physicians' beliefs shape reality, as the above studies strongly
suggest, these "doctor beliefs" are capable independently of causing
great harm. This means that patients should carefully examine the beliefs of a doctor before affiliating with him or her. In my experience this
is not commonly done. Patients may be attentive to the doctor's credentials, postgraduate training, and years of experience, but rarely do
they go further to inquire about the physician's belief structure and the
effect it might have on their outcome.

How can this be done? One need not subject the doctor to a
lengthy interrogation or a detailed checklist of questions to determine
his or her belief structure. A simple but crucial question will suffice:
Does my doctor make me feel better or worse when I'm around him or her?
This is one of the simplest but most effective ways of penetrating the
belief structure of a physician.

The importance of this issue was brought home to me in a letter I
received from a woman with AIDS. She had contracted the disease
from her husband, and was being treated at monthly intervals by an expert in infectious diseases. The doctor was a stern, no-nonsense fellow
who fit the classic picture of the cool, dispassionate scientist. He believed in presenting a "realistic" picture to all his patients. He would re-
mind the woman on each visit that since AIDS is "uniformly fatal," it
was critical that she follow her treatment to the letter. The doctor's beliefs had devastating effects. She said,

> I began to realize my doctor doesn't *believe* I'm going to live. . . . It
> takes me two weeks to recover from a visit to him. He leaves me
> depressed and feeling sick. But after two weeks have passed, I al-
> ways begin to feel terrific. Then, when it's time to return for an
> appointment, a feeling of dread overwhelms me. I have to make

myself keep my appointment. After the visit the cycle repeats it-self. . . . Why do I feel like my own physician is *killing* me?

If the double-blind studies demonstrating the potency of the doc-tor's belief are valid, this doctor's behavior may be unethical: he may ac-tually be pushing his patient toward a negative outcome. But we must admit that this situation is very complex. Many physicians feel com-pelled to be totally factual with their patients, sometimes against their better judgment, because of the fear of legal recriminations. If they do not present a "realistic" picture, they may be sued for misleading a pa-tient and be judged guilty of misrepresentation. Without some change in the legal climate, it is doubtful that most doctors will become coura-geous enough to intentionally use belief therapeutically, in spite of the fact that they may honor the evidence of its power to heal.

THE CONNECTION BETWEEN
PRAYER AND BELIEF

The power of the physician's belief system to shape the patient's responses to therapy is akin to prayer. Both prayer and belief are nonlocal manifestations of consciousness, because both can operate at a distance, sometimes outside the patient's awareness. Both affirm that "it's not all physical," and both can be used adjunctively with other forms of therapy.

How can a physician who is genuinely and honestly skeptical about a therapy use his or her beliefs positively for the good of the pa-tient? Perhaps the first rule should be never to select a therapy one doesn't believe in. When this isn't possible—when a last-ditch therapy is chosen in a near-hopeless situation, for example—the doctor should continue nonetheless to be as hopeful and open as possible under the circumstances. The goal should be never to obstruct healing by being unnecessarily pessimistic. And in addition to allowing their positive be-liefs about a particular therapy to flow freely, those physicians believing in prayer should actually employ it. If one is convinced that prayer works, *not* to use it is analogous to withholding a potent medication or surgical procedure.

THE SHAMAN AND THE INTERNIST

Because there may be no such thing as a *perfect* fit between the beliefs of a physician and a patient, two of the most valuable
qualities a physician can cultivate are those of flexibility and tolerance.
These capacities make it possible for a physician to honor a patient's
point of view, even though it may not be his or her own; and they per-
mit the physician to consider a variety of approaches to a particular
problem.

One of my most vivid lessons in flexibility in a healer began when
I received an unexpected phone call one day from Ken, a close friend.

"He's in pain, and he wants to see you," Ken said. "Look, he's really hurting. What do you mean, you're not sure you should treat him.
You're a *doctor*, aren't you?"

"Yes," I said. "But he's a *shaman*."

The shaman in question was Rolling Thunder, the legendary Native American healer and spiritual teacher from Nevada. He became famous in the 1970s when Doug Boyd featured him and his remarkable
healing powers in a book by the same name.[12] I had read the book and
was awed by Rolling Thunder's abilities. Like all shamans he apparently
could enter into the natural world experientially and manipulate it in
ways that were completely unexplainable by modern science.

He was in Dallas to give a series of lectures on shamanic healing
that Ken had helped arrange. All was not going well, however. Rolling
Thunder was scheduled to give a major lecture that evening, but he had
come down with a severe neck ache. He told Ken he wanted to see a
physician. Ken was worried that the lecture might have to be canceled,
and was scrambling to find a doctor who would see Rolling Thunder on
short notice.

I agreed to see him that afternoon, but was distinctly uncomfortable doing so because the situation was so utterly paradoxical. Why
would a powerful shaman, who seemed to have nothing in common
with the world of modern medicine, want to visit an internist for a neck
ache? Why should he not cure himself? Or why not see another
shaman, someone who shared his beliefs about healing? Why go outside his own system?

As the hour for Rolling Thunder's appointment neared, I found myself becoming increasingly anxious. What could I possibly say to this famous healer? If he could not cure his problem, what chance did I have to help?

At the appointed hour, I looked down the hall to see a nurse leading a colorful entourage of Native Americans all dressed in western wear, including black hats and silver-and-turquoise belts. Rolling Thunder had come with his friends, and the group was quite impressive. The nurse presented me with his patient chart (clinic rule: *Nobody* can see a physician without a chart!). The idea of a famous shaman with a medical chart seemed ludicrous. Then I glanced at the name on the chart and almost broke into laughter. He had been signed in as "Thunder, Rolling"—last name always first!

Thunder Comma Rolling and I exchanged pleasantries. I told him how much I had benefited from reading Boyd's book about him many years ago.

"They tell me it's good! Never read it myself," he said, smiling. "Guess I ought to someday."

I showed him into an examining room, while his friends sat in the waiting area. Rule number one: Take a history. "Why did you decide to come to see me?" I asked

"I've got a bad pain in my neck."

"Tell me about it."

"Every time I give talks they make me use a microphone. I stand up straight and move my neck forward to speak into it. It's not natural. It puts a strain on my neck and I always get this pain." He craned his neck forward to demonstrate the awkward position, and showed me the area where he hurt.

Rule number two: Do a physical exam. I could find nothing abnormal except for some hard, taut neck muscles that were in spasm and painful to touch.

"Let's go into my office and chat," I said. He followed me and we sat down. Our conversation began to flow freely. It drifted back to the book, to his life in Nevada, to the things he enjoyed, such as flying in small planes. All the while I was asking myself the best way to deal with his immediate problem.

Acting on a strong hunch, I finally decided to get down to business. "Rolling Thunder, what do you think about the use of drugs?"

"Why do you think I've come?"

He went on to explain his personal philosophy of healing. There is a time for the shaman's chants, prayers, and herbs, he said. There is also a place for a modern approach, including the use of synthetic chemical medications. A wise healer uses what works. He does not confine himself to a single methodology. All things considered, Rolling Thunder believed the use of drugs was the best treatment for his neck ache in this situation.

I went to the area where we kept sample medications and returned with two, a pain reliever and a muscle relaxant. I handed them to Rolling Thunder and he beamed.

"These will help me get through my talk tonight," he responded.

I accompanied him down the hall to meet his friends. On the way we passed Patrick, a vascular surgeon. Patrick was the only surgeon I knew who was a strict vegetarian.

"Patrick, I'd like you to meet my friend Rolling Thunder." The men shook hands.

"It's a pleasure to meet you," Patrick said. Rolling Thunder simply nodded. He seemed fascinated with Patrick. His eyes narrowed as he scrutinized him slowly from head to toe. After a few moments of deliberation, he said to Patrick, "Do you eat a lot of greens?"

Patrick was speechless as Rolling Thunder smiled and ambled down the hall.

The drugs worked. Rolling Thunder was in fine form at his lecture that night, speaking—through the microphone he despised—to a packed house.

Chapter 9

When Prayer Hurts: An Inquiry into "Black Prayer"

> It is held in most sacred traditions that virtually any capacity can be communicated without sensory cues. Such capacities . . . can be used destructively. The same religious traditions that celebrate metanormal transmission of illumined states also bear witness to communication abilities employed for egocentric, bullying, even monstrous purposes. There is a lore in virtually every religious culture about adepts who use their special powers . . . for selfish ends. This lore . . . is supported by modern research. . . .
>
> —Michael Murphy, *The Future of the Body*

During the drug trial of General Manuel Noriega in Miami, Florida, the jury was hopelessly deadlocked. Then they had a prayer session. The next morning they returned with a quick guilty verdict. Noriega's defense lawyers cried foul. They contended that the jurors were "improperly influenced" by the prayer, and that prayer unfairly led to their client's conviction. This was ironic, since Noriega claimed to have undergone a jail-house religious conversion himself, which presumably also involved prayer. Thus there are a few attorneys who, while not admitting that prayer can actually *harm*, seem to believe that it can at least *confuse*.[1]

145

Negative (sometimes called "black") prayer is the flip side of prayer as we generally think of it. In black prayer, rather than asking the Absolute to intercede benevolently in human affairs, one invokes the powers to cause harm or wreak havoc. Although this prompts several important questions about human nature and the nature of evil, that is not our focus here. We will instead examine whether or not there is any scientific evidence that human beings can use prayer to harm others. We will see that this possibility is supported not only by lore and legend, but by actual laboratory evidence as well.

Followers of Western religions tend erroneously to believe that sorcery, hexing, and cursing are engaged in only by "uncivilized" peoples. But these activities permeate all religions and cultures. "Many saintly curses would be right at home in the Bible," says John Carey, associate professor of Celtic languages and literature at Harvard University. Elisha, for example, caused forty-two children to be devoured by bears for making fun of his baldness (2 Kings 2:23–24). Reminiscent of the titanic power struggles between dueling shamans, the apostle Paul struck a sorcerer blind (Acts 13:11). And even Christ blasted an apparently innocent fig tree for not bearing fruit (Matthew 21:19, Mark 11:13–14, 20–22).[2]

What does science say about the possibility of negative distant phenomena? Its attitude is hardly cordial. Contemporary science largely rejects *all* action-at-a-distance, positive *and* negative. In his epochal book *The Golden Bough*, Sir James Frazer describes science's objections:

> [M]agic is a spurious system of natural law . . . it is a false science as well as an abortive art. . . . [C]ontagious magic commits the mistake of assuming that things which have once been in contact with each other are always in contact. . . . [Such beliefs are typical of] the crude intelligence not only of the savage, but [of] ignorant and dull-witted people everywhere.[3]

This attitude may sound paternalistic or even archaic, written as it was earlier in this century. But the prevailing attitude among most professional investigators has changed little since Frazer railed against "magic" and "savages" in 1922.

NEGATIVE INFLUENCES IN THE LABORATORY

If we suspend Frazer's verdict, what evidence can we find in support of negative distant influences? Let's take a look.

Olga Worrall: "I Refuse to Hurt Them"

Many healers who actually use prayer to help others will freely admit its potential for harm. Among them was the late Olga Worrall, the well-known psychic healer. Beverly Rubik, director of the Center for Frontier Sciences at Temple University, and physicist Elizabeth Rauscher, performed laboratory studies on Worrall, whose approach to healing was deeply spiritual and grounded in prayer. Rubik asked Worrall to interact with a suspension of bacteria, inhibiting or retarding their growth or actually killing them. Bacterial counts would then be made and compared to a control sample. Rubik could thus determine with great accuracy whether Worrall could exert a real effect or not on living organisms. Worrall strenuously objected. "I refuse to hurt them," she said. "I will only use my abilities for good." Honoring her wishes, Rubik modified the experiment in a way that enabled Worrall to use her powers positively. Two samples of bacteria would be exposed to the toxic effects of an antibacterial agent, and Worrall would "protect" one sample but not the other. The results showed that the "protected" bacteria indeed survived in greater numbers than the controls, at levels of great statistical significance.[4]

The Case of the Petrified Banana

Researcher Bernard Grad, who performed landmark experiments on reputed psychic healers at Canada's McGill University,[5] relates a story that suggests that certain people can generate extraordinarily negative effects on living entities. During the course of Grad's research, a man heard of his experiments and volunteered to be studied. He claimed he had the ability, using his hands, to cause an unusual reaction in certain living things such as fruit. He would hold a banana, for example, and focus on it in a specific way, whereupon it would begin to desiccate, blacken, and shrink. Not only would it become dry and change color, it would *petrify*. These changes were accelerated, occurring over a few hours, not at all like the normal changes that take place in fruit over days.

At one of his lectures, Grad was parenthetically discussing this strange event. He had retained one of the petrified bananas and had had it mounted on a key chain. He retrieved it from his pocket and banged it vigorously on the podium to demonstrate its hardness. I investigated it after the lecture and could hardly believe it: a miniature, rock-solid banana resembling marble.

Uri Geller's Surprise

Many years ago Zvi Bentwich, an internationally known Israeli researcher in the field of immunology, conducted tests on the famous psychic Uri Geller. Professor Bentwich relates the following events.[6]

Geller was widely accused of being a fraud. Bentwich's team designed a variety of sensitive laboratory tests to provide Geller a chance to demonstrate his psychic skills, while excluding chicanery and sleight-of-hand. In one particular experiment, Geller held his hands over a container of live sperm. His goal was to change their motility, their patterns of movement, as judged by microscopic examination. The experiment was arranged with proper controls, and any effect of heat from his hands was eliminated. When the "treated" sperm were promptly examined, the experimenters discovered they were completely *dead*, while the controls were normal. When the supernate, the fluid in which the dead sperm were contained, was collected and applied to normal sperm, there was no effect, which ruled out the possibility that Geller surreptitiously had applied a chemical of some sort that killed the sperm. Geller was reportedly very shaken by this sudden and unexpected glimpse into his capacity to cause harm. He had intended only to change the motility of the sperm, not *kill* them. His capacity to cause harm resembles negative effects of prayer, as we shall see.

Black Thumbs, Green Thumbs

Controlled laboratory experiments show that ordinary people can use their minds either to inhibit *or* promote the growth of microorganisms.[7] These effects occur when the "influencer" is from a yard and a half to fifteen miles away from the microorganisms.[8] These studies may support the folk idea that some people seem naturally to have "bad vibes" that sabotage the growth of their houseplants, flowers, and so on—the "black thumb" phenomenon. We also recognize the opposite—the "green thumb" effect—in which plants seem to thrive in the presence of some people. As an example of someone who seemed capable of affecting living things positively at the genetic level, researcher Daniel J. Benor cites Luther Burbank, "who appeared to have a paranormal ability to produce new strains of plants, developing more than 800 new varieties in his lifetime—an unmatched record in horticulture."[9] Burbank seemed convinced that humans and plants can interact. He once remarked, "Plants are as responsive to thought as children."[10]

These studies should give us pause. If people can *retard* or *inhibit* the growth of microorganisms—with which we share many identical biochemical processes—why should these negative influences not extend to humans?

Hypnosis at a Distance

The history of hypnosis is richly peppered with evidence suggesting that it is possible for one person to affect the behavior of a distant individual without the "receiver's" awareness that the effort is taking place. In some of these cases, the hypnotist seems almost to be toying with the subject. Consider this anecdote from the late 1800s. One day the famous physician and hypnotist Charles Richet was sitting in the dining room of Beaujon Hospital with his colleague Landusi. Richet declared that he could put one of his patients to sleep at a distance and compel her to come to the dining room solely by an act of his will. After ten minutes had elapsed, however, nobody came. Richet and Landusi considered the experiment a failure—until a few minutes later, when someone came to the dining room to announce that a sleeping patient was found roaming the corridors of the hospital, searching for Dr. Richet, whom she could not find.[11]

Similar experiments were performed around the same time in Le Havre, by the well-known psychiatrist Pierre Janet[12]; and in the 1930s by the prominent Russian researchers Vasiliev, Platonov, Bekhterev, Dubrovsky, and Tomashevsky.[13]

These findings, many of which were conducted in elaborate laboratory settings, are sobering. They suggest strongly that we have the capacity to radically alter the behavior of distant individuals, outside their awareness, possibly for harm.

EVIDENCE FROM ANTHROPOLOGY

Because anthropologists study cultures in which distant hexing is said to abound, I felt they should know whether these events really happen or not. For many years, whenever I got the chance, I asked them about these possibilities. Invariably their answer was, "No, of course they don't really occur," or some variation thereof. Most seemed decidedly uncomfortable every time I brought up the question, and eventually I decided they simply did not want to discuss the issue.[14]

I let the question drop until I found myself at a conference sitting across a dinner table from Professor Michael Harner, the noted anthropologist and authority on shamanism. I realized I had a chance to inquire from a genuine scholar. Harner had spent years doing fieldwork studying the Jivaro Indians, who lived near the headwaters of the Amazon. During these visits he learned their language, entered their culture, and became intimately aware of the various aspects of Jivaro daily life.

"Dr. Harner, have you ever met shamans who could hex someone at a distance without the victim knowing about it?" I asked.

"In Jivaro culture distant hexing is taken for granted," Harner said without hesitation. "Many of the shamans I've studied on the Amazon have claimed to be very good at it. I have no reason to disbelieve them."

"Why do they hex people at a distance?" I asked. "Why not person-to-person, as in voodoo?"

"Their rationale is simple," Harner responded. "If the victim is unaware he's being hexed, he won't take measures to counteract the hex or take revenge on the shaman or try actually to kill him. As an added safety measure, the Jivaro shamans perform distant hexing as a team of two or three, not alone. If the victim tries to get even, there's safety in numbers. Distant hexing is really a security measure."[15]

Distant hexing or negative prayer are not to be confused with voodoo. In voodoo the sorcerer typically manipulates the victim's symbolic image, whether it is a doll, the person's clothing, body exuviae, hair, nail parings, dirt from the victim's tracks, or a photograph. Then, according to the physiologist Walter Cannon, the subject is intentionally made *aware* that he has been hexed.[16] The victim's awareness of the curse is the foundation on which the hex rests. Realizing he is cursed, he lives out his fate and cooperates with the hex by dying. The villagers also realize what is taking place and behave toward the victim as if he is actually going to die, which hastens his demise.[17]

Voodoo-type hexing is a *local* happening. That is, it takes place in a particular point in space and time, in the here-and-now experience of the victim and his or her acquaintances. Negative prayer is not a local but a *nonlocal* event, being initiated at a distance from the recipient, outside his or her awareness. Voodoo is mediated by sensory mechanisms—hearing, speaking, visual cues, touch, and so on. In distant hexing or negative prayer, the victim is totally unaware of the curse and has no sensory contact with the perpetrator. Since there are no known physical mechanisms whereby the negative prayer or hex could be transmitted, it is scientifically impossible for such an event to happen. This is probably the major reason why academic anthropologists are reluctant to study or even report such phenomena.

Holger Kalweit, a German ethnologist who has studied shamanism in Hawaii, the American Southwest, Mexico, and Tibet, has provided an expert view of the fascinating dark side of shamanism in his book *Shamans, Healers, and Medicine Men*.[18] In Kalweit's view the effects of black magic—"maleficent thoughts that are transferred onto an enemy"—depend on three underlying principles: 1. "the principle of a telepathic communication network and the connection of all people through a telepathic link . . . common to all nature peoples"; 2. the understanding that "the universe is . . . a pulsating unity to which

everyone, especially medicine persons, can open themselves"; and 3.
"the principle of empathic attunement—as it existed in the primordial
time when there was communication with all living beings, including
stones, plants, and even heaven and earth." *These are the same principles
we have seen already to underlie the loving, benevolent use of prayer.*

In his book *Coyote On a Wounded Planet*, Neal Claremon shows
how these principles come together to influence all aspects of life, particularly our relationships with others, for either good or ill. As he
makes clear, we do not have to belong to native cultures or be shamans
for these states of consciousness to affect us; *they operate at deep levels,
whether we know it or not.*[19]

Kalweit cites an intriguing example of how anger and negative
thoughts can get out of hand and harm an innocent person at a distance:

> John Quinn of the Tenino tribe of Oregon was accused by his
> tribal brothers of committing three murders. For only an instant,
> Quinn harbored an evil thought against one of the men charging
> him. His helping spirit immediately understood this thought as an
> order to kill this individual. The spirit charged off at full speed to
> carry out this wish, but collided with an innocent young girl who
> happened to be passing by the door. Quinn was not aware of this.
> Before he or any other shaman could come to her aid, the girl
> died.[20]

In another example, a man with shamanic power used it for retri-
bution:

> Billy, an Australian shepherd near Kijuliji Station, possessed an
> extraordinary ability to concentrate his thoughts. He was not per-
> mitted to eat his meals in the kitchen of the station with the
> whites, but was given his food to eat outside alone. When he got
> up late one morning, his white boss threw his food onto the
> garbage heap. Billy walked silently back to his camp, but only
> after thinking his *'maulwa*, or cord, out of his body and knotting it
> into a kind of net. He proceeded to throw it over the doors and
> windows of the boss's house, and dragged the cord behind him as
> he walked back to camp. He then unleashed his helping totem,

lightning, which struck the house and set it on fire. When the cook tried to put out the cookstove with water, Billy "sung" the water into kerosene, which made things worse.[21]

Can we study these events in the laboratory? Anthropologist Joan Halifax is skeptical. She states, "Although [these hexing] situations seem quite fantastic, . . . they certainly deserve systematic exploration *in the field*. I emphasize field research. . . . [I]t is highly improbable, if not absurd, to attempt to replicate such experiences in the laboratory."[22]

One problem with studying these phenomena in the laboratory is that if hexing worked, subjects might die. A professor who taught a course called "Parapsychology of the Occult" actually took this risk. One of his students claimed he had the ability to perform hex deaths. For his term paper, he wanted to demonstrate this talent. The professor agreed. "[But] . . . we couldn't have him try to kill just anyone—that wouldn't be fair or nice," the professor said. "So we agreed that he would attempt by hex death to kill me." The professor left a sealed envelope with the registrar, on which he wrote, "Open this upon my death if it occurs within the next year." Inside the envelope a note instructed the registrar to give the student an "A" if the professor died. The student agreed that if the professor did not die, he would receive an "F." The student flunked. Said the professor, "I think there are a lot of people around who would be willing to be targets for people who claim they can perform hex deaths, myself included . . . we can test [this hypothesis]."[23]

THE "DEATH PRAYER"

In 1917 psychologist Max Freedom Long arrived in Hawaii and took a job as a teacher in the area near the Kilauea volcano. He had been interested in comparative religion all his life. This set the stage for his fascination with the native magicians, the *kahunas*, or "Keepers of the Secret," whose lore he managed to penetrate with great effort.[24]

Long devoted intensive study to kahuna magic and came away with not only respect but admiration for it. "[I]f we can learn to use it as did the native magicians of Polynesia . . . ," he said, "[it] bids fair to change the world."[25] He was fascinated in particular with *ana-ana*, Hawaiian for the "death prayer."

He discovered that in the kahuna tradition of Polynesia, which spread to the Hawaiian Islands, the "death prayer" had a redeeming social value. As he describes its function,

> The kahunas taught . . . the people to live without hurting others. Those who willfully hurt others were considered worthy of death, and were frequently punished with the death prayer. It was the means of developing in Polynesia the most friendly and considerate people in the entire world. All the early explorers marveled at this and mentioned it in their writings without exception.[26]

The kahunas were prescient psychologists. They believed that each individual had two souls or spirits instead of one.[27] These corresponded roughly to the unconscious and the conscious parts of the mind. Long observes that the early missionaries thought the idea of two souls "a most droll and idiotic concept, worthy only of heathens and savages. To them, man had but one soul, and their job was to save it if possible."[28] The idea that the human mind might have composite parts simply did not occur to the missionaries. This was 1820, a half century before Freud.

This psychological topography is what made the death prayer possible. The kahunas realized—as we in the West would later acknowledge—that the unconscious mind is highly susceptible to suggestion, even if the suggestion is absurd and illogical. This susceptibility allowed the "death influence" to be implanted in the unconscious, causing the victim to die.

The weak spot in the armor of the unconscious that allowed the insertion of the fatal influence was usually *guilt*. Long emphasizes its key role in mediating death by prayer: guilt was "the secret and greatly important thing known to the kahunas, but only faintly glimpsed and entirely misunderstood by religionists around the world."[29] An individual who possessed a deep sense of guilt for some actual or imaginary sin could be attacked by a spirit bent on punishing or killing him. The unconscious, convinced of its unworthiness, would meekly accept the attack because of its conviction that it *deserved* to be punished.

So far this may sound like conventional voodoo, in which the victim's death occurs as a result of suggestion and cooperation with the known hex. But unlike voodoo the death prayer is mediated nonlocally at a distance, completely outside the victim's awareness, in the absence of any sensory cues or information delivered to him or her. Long recognized the uniqueness of this feature and emphasized it repeatedly. "None of the usual explanations of the 'death prayer,' such as the use of a mysterious poison or of 'dying of superstition' were true," he says. "Almost never did the victim know that he was about to be killed by magic."[30]

The victim's symptoms followed a typical pattern. First the feet would "go to sleep," then the prickling numbness would creep slowly upward to the level of the waist. This would be accompanied by a "slow paralysis" of the lower limbs. These symptoms would eventually be followed by a general collapse and death.[31]

IS THE UNIVERSE CONTAGIOUS?

Earlier we noted Sir James Frazer's remark that, "[C]ontagious magic commits the mistake of assuming that *things which have once been in contact with each other are always in contact*" [emphasis added]. Ironically, as we have already noted, recent advances in the field of modern quantum mechanics demonstrate that the phenomenon that so thoroughly repulsed Sir James actually exists at the subatomic level. As a result of a development called Bell's theorem, and the many subsequent experiments relating to it, physicists now maintain that once subatomic particles have been in contact, they always in some sense remain connected; and that a change in one creates a simultaneous change in the other, even if they are separated to the opposite ends of the universe. "Contagious magic" seems to be woven into the fabric of the universe!

This point deserves emphasis. Physicist Nick Herbert, an authority on the implications of Bell's theorem, describes these developments in his book *Quantum Reality*:

> Despite physicists' traditional rejection of non-local interaction, despite the fact that all known forces are incontestably local, despite Einstein's prohibition against superluminal [faster-than-light]

connections, . . . Bell maintains that the world is filled with innumerable non-local influences. Furthermore, these unmediated connections are present not only in rare and exotic circumstances, but underlie all the events of everyday life. Non-local connections are ubiquitous because reality itself is non-local.[32]

Could humans be joined in much the same eerie way that subatomic particles are connected, and could this connectedness make possible negative prayer and distant hexing? Certainly Bell's theorem *does not prove* that these events occur, or even that they are possible; indeed there is robust debate among anthropologists whether they exist at all, as we've noted. Moreover Bell's theorem deals with invisible subatomic particles, not humans—although physicist Herbert has offered a proof that shows that the theorem is applicable not only to the invisible world of quantum events, but to our large-scale, familiar world as well. Inserting the concept of nonlocality into this debate might be valuable—for if anthropologists and other investigators were aware that the *principle* of nonlocality is today a legitimate part of modern physics, our most accurate science, perhaps this would encourage them to keep an open mind about these strange reports.

Frazer again: "[C]ontagious magic commits the mistake of assuming that things which have once been in contact with each other are always in contact." But there is no "mistake" as Frazer thought, since this is the way the universe operates at the subatomic level. *Whether this makes God the ultimate practitioner of contagious magic is an interesting question.*

IS ONLY CARING CONTAGIOUS?

Daniel J. Benor, whose English literature survey of psychic healing is included in Appendix 1, was once challenged by a questioner who felt that if prayer had positive effects on humans, it also might have negative influences. Benor's response:

> Your concern is one that is shared by most people who hear about psychic healing. They say if a healer can think positive changes into me, can he not also think negative changes into me? The reports of both the healers and the healees have consistently been in

the positive direction, that negative effects do not occur. I . . . have reviewed the literature exhaustively. The only negative effects that are reported are of pain being eliminated when people were concerned that perhaps they ought to have some pain to let them know whether their illness was progressing or not progressing. And that was just a conjecture. No one has come up with a case in which the elimination of pain proved to be dangerous. There have been reports of healers actually bringing about the demise of animals, in one case a rat, in another case a cow. . . . Bacteria have been killed by healers . . . it is hard to know what to make of those isolated reports.[33]

A South African study suggests that there might be some benevolent force in the universe insuring only positive expressions of prayer, while guarding against its negative use. In this study a healer tried to influence the growth of tumors in thirty mice. While attempts to *decrease* the size of the tumors were highly successful, the healer was unable to *increase* the size.[34]

There are some constant features of telesomatic cases (see chapter 2) that also suggest an inherent benignity to distant events. These happenings usually take place between people who share empathic, loving bonds—parents and children, spouses, siblings, lovers. And even though noxious or painful symptoms or sensations are "transmitted," these feelings usually serve a benevolent or higher purpose—as when a mother experiences a suffocating feeling and "just knows" her infant has fallen into the swimming pool, and rushes home to save her.

This leads many people to believe that if caring, compassion, love, and empathy are the "sparks" that bridge the gap between distant people, prayer never hurts. I understand why people want this to be true. There is something in the human psyche that hates ambiguity, that wants things to be clear, and that wants prayer to be helpful and benign but never harmful. I too would like to believe there is a protective, benevolent quality in the world that guards against the willful infliction of harm on a distant person through prayer. But after examining the ethnographic and experimental evidence, I believe we must come to grips with the possibility that negative prayer is real.

In all the world, I know of no therapies that are totally free of side effects. Physicians inadvertently kill tens of thousands of people annually via the unanticipated side effects of drugs and surgical procedures. All types of healers of whom I am aware also manage to harm people, sometimes gravely. Acupuncture needles have caused bloodstream infections and endocarditis, infection of the heart's valves; herbs of a great variety, widely claimed to be free of side effects because they are "natural," have caused reactions ranging from skin rashes to anaphylactic shock; "harmless" spinal manipulation has caused quadriplegia. So it may be with prayer: although its potential for healing is immense, there is a dark side, which not even its connection with the Divine can erase. Why should it? The Divine, after all, contains a dark side: even Lucifer once resided in heaven.

As a physician I find it wise to ask of any therapy at the outset: What is the downside? What are the side effects? What is the potential for harm? I would ask these questions of prayer. Too often we have been regaled with promises of breakthroughs and miracle cures, later to be disappointed as we discover the therapy's negative aspects. We can be enthusiastic about the positive effects of prayer—as we are justified in being—but we need not be Pollyanas.

PART 3

THE EVIDENCE

Chapter 10

God in the Laboratory

> We attend our lodges, encounter groups, holistic health,
> martial arts, and religious group meetings on the week-
> ends or in the evenings, and the following morning put
> on our working clothes to return to strictly analytical, in-
> creasingly digital, virtually impersonal manipulation of
> our business or professional responsibilities. And all the
> while, well beneath our starched collars or laboratory
> coats, frail and timid vestiges of our spiritual selves con-
> tinue to dream, to hope, to love, and to pray.
>
> At the risk of sounding like *Star Trek*'s Mr. Spock, is
> it logical for humans to indulge in wishing, or praying, or
> loving, yet to doubt the efficacy of such activities? Or if
> their empirical effectiveness is acknowledged, why should
> such phenomena be exempt from scientific study, or from
> systematic application in our pragmatic or scholarly areas
> of activity? Why cannot our mystical and mental selves
> coexist in both practical and spiritual affairs; indeed, why
> can they not simply coalesce?
>
> —Robert G. Jahn and Brenda J. Dunne,
> *Margins of Reality*

In the spring of 1992, I was invited to participate in a
health conference in Israel on the shores of the Dead Sea. How ironic, I
thought, discussing *health* on the banks of a *dead* body of water—just
the sort of paradoxes that abound in the Middle East! It was my first
visit to that part of the world, and I was deeply impressed by the experience. It is not difficult to be moved by desert surroundings, particularly

this one, where prophets and potentates have railed at one another for millennia, where three of the world's great religions were born, and where some of the most savage wars known to humankind have raged.

Following the conference I went to Jerusalem. I wanted especially to visit the *Kotel*, the Western Wall, often referred to as the Wailing Wall because Jews traditionally go there to mourn the destruction of their Temple. King Solomon, believed to have written the Books of Proverbs, Ecclesiastes, and the Song of Songs, originally built the Temple about 950 B.C. in what frequently is referred to as Israel's Golden Era. The Wailing Wall was built by Herod the Great in 20 B.C. to support the Temple's esplanade. After an extended siege of Jerusalem in A.D. 70, the Roman general Titus breached the city wall and destroyed the Temple. The Wailing Wall remained. It is a vivid reminder to all Jews of their rich history and is one of the most famous sites in all of Israel. At all hours one can see Hasidic Jews in their distinctive black clothes, bobbing to and fro before the wall's massive stones, as they translate the rhythms of their prayers into bodily movements.

Though I am not Jewish, I nonetheless found myself drawn toward the wall with the Hasidim. Standing quietly alongside them, I noticed that the cracks between the gigantic stones were crammed with scraps of paper on which prayers had been written. Wanting to participate in this ancient ritual, I pulled a bit of paper from my pocket and stood poised, pen in hand, prepared to write my special prayer. But nothing would come. Even though I was surrounded by praying people, I literally could think of nothing that needed praying for. Everything at that moment seemed perfectly right just as it was. The only thing I could think of was: *I want to know the truth*.

Finally I folded my blank scrap of paper, inserted it in a cranny along with thousands of written entreaties, and silently walked away. As I left, an image of a different kind of wall entered my mind—a vision of a time when science was just beginning.

EARLY SCIENCE AND THE WALL OF TRUTH

In sixteenth-century Europe, as philosopher Jacob Needleman describes in *A Sense of the Cosmos*,[1] the church was the ultimate arbiter of reality, defining the workings of the world for everyone. Science—although the word did not exist then—arose in opposition to this custom; Galileo (1564–1642), condemned by the church to spend the last years of his life under house arrest, is perhaps the best-known example. What were these early scientists like? They were people who above all wanted a direct, unmediated encounter with reality, a personal experience in which no authority or dogma blocked their approach. In Needleman's graphic metaphor, these early scientists *went to the wall of truth*, where they confronted the world alone, and invited the universe to reveal itself through their primitive experiments.

This image of the early scientists' wall of truth seemed literal and concrete as I left the Wailing Wall in Jerusalem's Old City, and it had particular meaning for me. At the time I was working on this book about prayer, and I was struggling with the question of whether it was *desirable* to study prayer scientifically. My experience at the Wailing Wall left me with the feeling not only that it *could* be studied, but that it *should* be. Not everyone agrees.

WHY PEOPLE OBJECT TO STUDYING PRAYER SCIENTIFICALLY

Unlike his native counterpart, to whom seeking knowledge is a sacred endeavor, the Western scientist treats any such feelings as a contaminant and a potential vitiation of scientific objectivity. . . . "the need to desacralize [the world is] a defense . . . against being flooded by emotion, especially the emotions of humility, reverence, mystery, wonder, and awe."

—Willis W. Harman[2]

More people than ever before are becoming convinced that some things should be off limits to science, that the scientist's wall of truth should extend only so far. They believe that science debases and violates whatever it touches. It is not difficult to see where this belief comes from. Prominent scientists state routinely that nothing in nature is sacred. They confidently assure us that the world is drifting along purposelessly, that it is utterly devoid of meaning, and that it is nothing more than inanimate matter in motion. Since no harm can be done to the inanimate, any method of investigation is justified.

English philosopher Francis Bacon (1561–1626) was a pivotal figure in the development of this attitude. Bacon strongly believed, in keeping with the biblical imperative, that it was human destiny to conquer nature and exercise dominion over it. By the end of the seventeenth century, in keeping with Bacon's vision, going to the wall of truth in science no longer involved veneration and a sacred regard for truth's objects.

The negative impact of this soulless approach persists to this day and has created a huge public relations problem for science. Many people believe that the general heartlessness of science is directly responsible for many global problems, such as pollution and environmental degradation of all sorts. When it comes to the question of investigating prayer scientifically, these same folks react predictably. They want nothing to do with the scientific method, and react with horror at the prospect that something Divine would be debased by the soiled hands and hard hearts of scientists.

To be sure, prayer does not need science to legitimize or justify it. Even so, I believe that if science *can* demonstrate the potency of prayer, people who pray are likely to feel empowered and validated in their beliefs as a result. Furthermore using science does not always require that we "put nature on the rack" and torture her to reveal her secrets, to use Bacon's images. Instead we can *honor* what is being investigated and approach it with respect and reverence. From this point of view, investigating prayer does not imply "bringing God into the laboratory," but "bringing the laboratory to God," requesting and inviting the Universe to reveal its workings.

When I began my search several years ago for empirical evidence for prayer's effectiveness, I naively believed that the organized religions would be delighted with experiments showing that prayer works. I came across work done by the Spindrift organization (see chapter 5), which strongly suggests that prayer can actually change the physical world. The Spindrift scientists were affiliated with the Christian Science church, and some were actually credentialed healers. They were delighted with their empirical studies. Here is a laboratory test, they

said, that can demonstrate not only the power of prayer, but whether or
not any individual healer has the talent to heal. The church did not
share their enthusiasm, but reacted instead with horror. They charged
the Spindrift investigators with heresy, stating that it was incorrect to
"bring God into the laboratory," and stripped one of the primary investigators of his credentials as a healer. Clearly the objections to scientific
research on prayer do not come only from orthodox scientists.

These objections against studying prayer empirically, coming
from both scientists and religionists, seem terribly *presumptuous*. How
can we conceivably know the mind of the Almighty? Because we can't,
we cannot say what the Absolute prefers and dislikes. For all we know,
God may take sheer delight in being probed scientifically, in being
tested experimentally.

In spite of these objections, more and more scientists are beginning to agree that prayer *should* be tested experimentally. One of the
premier laboratories to study the actions of consciousness is the Princeton Engineering Anomalies Research (PEAR) program headed by
Robert G. Jahn, former dean of engineering at Princeton University,
and his colleagues, including Brenda J. Dunne and Roger Nelson. Jahn
and Dunne have long been aware of the philosophical and spiritual implications of their work. They believe religion could benefit from the
scientific study of prayer. Their enlightened attitude could serve as an
imprimatur for this entire book:

> Virtually all contemporary religions, like most of their predeces-
> sors, trade heavily on such mystical attitudes and activities as faith,
> hope, love, prayer, and sacrifice. Research results . . . may add an-
> other perspective to such elusive metaphysical concepts. Indeed,
> the relevance and vitality of theology in an increasingly analytical
> and technological age might well benefit from its own appropriate
> forms of scientific research, in much the same way that modern
> diagnostic and computational techniques have advanced factual
> comprehension and even aesthetic appreciation in such tradition-
> ally impressionistic fields as art, music, and literature. . . . [3]

In the end whether or not prayer can be proved experimentally
does not depend on anyone's *opinion* on the matter. The question can

only be settled by actually performing experiments to see whether or not there is an effect that comes through under laboratory conditions.

IS PRAYER A PLACEBO?

Skeptics say there is no reason to study prayer because basically there is nothing *to* study. Prayer simply does not work; any effects we observe are due only to suggestion—the famous placebo response. The word *placebo*, derived from Latin words meaning "I shall please," is "a harmless, unmedicated preparation given as a medicine to a patient merely to humor him."[4]

Is prayer a placebo? We can find at least three answers to this important question.

1. *Prayer can act as a placebo.* A person who merely knows that he or she is being prayed for can mobilize healing energies that can be awesomely potent. When this happens the effects of prayer are originating within the patient, not without. Scientists working in the new field of psychoneuroimmunology have demonstrated the existence of intimate links between the parts of the brain concerned with thought and emotion, and the neurological and immune systems.[5] Based on these discoveries, we know beyond doubt that thought can become biology—including the thought that one is being prayed for.

2. *Prayer can be intrinsically harmful.* The possibility that prayer can be harmful is almost never considered because true believers think prayer is always helpful, and skeptics are convinced it is uniformly worthless. But if the effects of suggestion in prayer are real—the placebo response—we should automatically propose harmful effects of prayer, because suggestion is a two-edged sword: it can be either positive or negative.

As we have seen in chapter 9, prayer can exert harm in two ways. One way is via negative placebo effects, which is the same as negative suggestion.[6] Knowing that negative prayer is being directed toward him, the victim can "live out" the harmful effects and actually die. The second way prayer can cause harm is by being used *nonlocally*, at a distance, even when the "receiver" is completely unaware that the attempt is being made—a phenomenon that cannot in principle be explained by suggestion or placebo effects.

3. *Prayer can be intrinsically helpful.* This is a way of saying that prayer works positively, of itself, and that its beneficial power is not due entirely to suggestion and the placebo response. This does not mean that placebo or suggestion effects are never involved in prayer; they can *always* be a factor when a person prays for himself or when he realizes another is trying to help—whether the helper is employing a drug, a surgical procedure, prayer, or something else.

Evidence is abundant for an intrinsic, positive effect of prayer not only in humans but in mice, chicks, enzymes, fungi, yeast, bacteria, and cells of various sorts (see Appendix 1). We cannot dismiss these outcomes as being due to suggestion or placebo effects, since these so-called lower forms of life do not think in any conventional sense and are presumably not susceptible to suggestion.

But even in experiments involving humans, as we shall see, it has been possible to use prayer, imagery, and other types of influence without the subjects' awareness—thus eliminating by and large the effects of suggestion. The scientific evidence suggests—overwhelmingly, in my opinion—that the effects of prayer are not due entirely to placebo effects. *But,* I would ask, *even if they were, what would it matter?* Suppose a cancer disappears and it can be proved beyond doubt that its disappearance was due "just" to placebo effects and suggestion? The cure would be no less real nor less appreciated by the patient.

Skeptics admit that disease does occasionally go away when someone prays, but they are quick to add that this does not mean that prayer *caused* the cure. It "just happened" that the two events—the use of prayer and the disappearance of the cancer—occurred in sequence. Coincidence, they say, not causality, was involved. Again, it hardly matters to the patient. He or she is content to let the skeptics and true believers argue over whether correlation or actual causation was involved.

Yet from another perspective it matters *immensely* whether or not prayer actually works in health problems. The answers we give to the questions surrounding prayer have the greatest importance for our understanding of our place in the world, our relationship to the Absolute, the nature of human consciousness, our origins and destiny. That is why, I maintain, the scientific studies of spiritual healing are crucial: They can help us find answers to the great questions of life.

Chapter 11

Prayer and Healing: Reviewing the Research

> If there is any primary rule of science, it is . . . acceptance of the obligation to acknowledge and describe all of reality, all that exists, everything that is the case. . . . It must accept within its jurisdiction even that which it cannot understand, explain, that for which no theory exists, that which cannot be measured, predicted, controlled, or ordered. . . . It includes all levels or stages of knowledge, including the inchoate, . . . knowledge of low reliability, . . . and subjective experience.
>
> —Abraham Maslow

This chapter takes a hard look at the research that has been done on the efficacy of prayer in healing. By trying to walk a fine line between a lengthy review and a trivialized summary, I have struggled mightily to make this section succinct yet explanatory. This chapter should give you a flavor of what the studies look and feel like, and help you to make up your own mind about the evidence.

THE HUMAN STUDIES

Scientists have sought evidence for prayer's power for over a century. They looked first at human beings for proof, and so shall we.

Prayer for Kings and Clergy: The First Study

Sir Francis Galton, the eminent English scientist, writer, and pioneer in eugenics, made perhaps the first objective inquiry into the efficacy of prayer, published in the *Fortnightly Review* in 1872.[1]

Galton reveals that he undertook his study "for the satisfaction of [his] own conscience." For him the most persuasive reason to believe that prayer works is the indisputable fact that everyone uses it, pagans and orthodox believers alike. If prayer is not efficacious, why would it be universal? Or, Galton asks, could this be evidence of "the universal tendency of man to gross incredulity"?

"Many persons of high intellectual gifts and critical minds," Galton observed, "look upon it as an axiomatic certainty that they possess this power [of prayer], although it is impossible for them to establish any scientific criterion. . . . " In keeping with this skeptical view, he was unable to discover a single example "in which a medical man of any repute has attributed recovery to the influence of prayer." Surely this "eloquence of silence" on the part of physicians was significant. "Had prayers for the sick any notable effect, it is incredible but that the doctors, who are always on the watch for such things, should have observed it, and added their influence to that of the priests toward obtaining them for every sick man." It is not just doctors who were unaware of an effect of prayer; other types of scientific observers were equally mute on the subject. "There is not a single instance, to my knowledge, in which papers read before statistical societies have recognised the agency of prayer either on disease or on anything else."

Setting these misgivings aside, Galton resorted to statistical comparisons to decide if prayer works. He compared the length of life of clergy to that of "materialistic" people. If prayer promotes longevity, he reasoned, then clergy should live longer, being the most "prayerful class" of all and among the most prayed for. Galton selected one other group for comparison, whose health and longevity were much prayed for: sovereign heads of state. "The public prayer for the sovereign of every state, Protestant and Catholic, is and has been in the spirit of our own, 'Grant her in health long to live,'" he observed.

Galton found that while clergy as a whole lived slightly longer than doctors and lawyers in general, when the longevity of *eminent* clergy was compared to that of *eminent* doctors and lawyers, the clergy were the *shortest* lived of the three groups.[2] Neither did prayer protect heads of state: "Sovereigns are literally the shortest lived of all who have the advantage of affluence."

Galton deserves credit for supposing that prayer is amenable to empirical scrutiny, but researchers today would immediately spot several problems with his study. It is plagued with assumptions and design flaws typical of retrospective analyses. Galton tried to grapple with some of these. He acknowledged that his comparisons might not be valid—for example, royal life might be inherently unhealthy and "more fatal" than other types of existence. He admitted that prayer might actually neutralize some of these noxious effects, and thus be efficacious after all—that is, although sovereigns lived shorter lives, their lives would be shorter still if they went unprayed for—but he eventually dismissed these mitigating considerations as a "very questionable hypothesis."

In his book *Science and Providence*, John Polkinghorne, dean and chaplain of Trinity Hall, Cambridge, and a fellow of the Royal Society and former professor of mathematical physics at Cambridge University, reviewed Galton's unflattering findings about prayer. He suggests some factors Galton failed to consider. For instance, Polkinghorne notes that one of the reasons sovereigns lived shorter lives in spite of having access to good nourishment and housing may have been that they were exposed to one of the greatest hazards of the day—the continual ministrations of the medical profession![3]

Galton acknowledges that praying may make a person *feel* better. After all, the urge to "pour out the feelings in sound is not peculiar to man" but is universal, existing even in animals. For example, he describes how the hare screams just before being overtaken by the greyhound. So too does "any mother that has lost her young, and wanders about moaning and looking piteously for sympathy . . . which prompts men to pray in articulate words." Lamentations during moments of distress and terror thus permeate the animal world; it is only man's "superior intellectual powers" that distinguish his cries, in the form of prayer, from those of other creatures.

Writing in exalted prose—the kind of writing that unfortunately has vanished from scientific journals—Galton in the end affirms the value of prayer. Although there is no empirical evidence that it works, this is no reason to abandon it. In spite of science's negative verdict, prayer is good for its own sake. "A confident sense of communion with God must necessarily rejoice and strengthen the heart, and divert it from petty cares," he says. Those who believe in prayer

> can dwell on the undoubted fact, that there exists a solidarity between themselves and what surrounds them . . . that they are descended from an endless past, that they have a brotherhood with all that is, and have each his own share of responsibility in the parentage of an endless future. . . . [This] great idea . . . is quite powerful . . . and [can] give serenity during the trials of life and in the shadow of approaching death.[4]

Praying for a Son

Rupert Sheldrake, the Cambridge-trained plant biologist who is well known for his theory of morphogenetic fields and formative causation, examined the effects of prayer in India in a study that, like Galton's, is a retrospective analysis.[5] Most people in India want to have sons rather than daughters, and they incessantly go to temples to ask holy men to bless their marriage so they can have a son. A tremendous amount of psychological energy and praying goes into this effort. Sheldrake examined statistics of live male births in India and compared them to England, where the preference for sons is not as strong. He found that in *both* England and India, there are about 106 males to 100 females—just as in almost every other country. "If this enormous amount of psychic effort and praying and blessings of holy men . . . were working, you would expect on average the percentage of live male births to be higher," Sheldrake states.

The Redlands Experiment

One of the earliest attempts in this century to study prayer scientifically was the Prayer Experiment begun at the University of Redlands in Redlands, California, in September 1951. This experiment was popularized in a widely read book, *Prayer Can Change Your*

Life, by Dr. William R. Parker and Elaine St. Johns.[6] The test group included forty-five volunteers, aged twenty-two to sixty. One-third of these were university students and two-thirds were housewives, teachers, businessmen, and others from the surrounding community. The volunteers brought a variety of problems to the study. They included depression and feeling "inactive and worn out," or "extinguished." Some had "exaggerated fears, lengthened shadows of the worry and depression which dogs us all from time to time." Others belonged to "that 50 to 75 per cent who seek medical treatment when there is nothing organically wrong."

Patients were divided into three groups of fifteen. Group I was the "Just-Plain-Psychology" group. No mention of religion was made during their therapy. Each of these persons had professed a preference for this type of treatment, or had been recommended for psychotherapy by their physicians.

Group II—the "Just-Plain-Prayer" group—prayed for themselves every night before retiring for the nine months of the experiment. They were faithful, practicing Christians who had immense confidence in prayer, and who believed psychological counseling unnecessary. They believed they knew how to pray well, and no further techniques in prayer were offered to them. The object of their prayers was to eradicate the problems at hand, whether emotional or physical ills.

Group III—the "Prayer Therapy Group"—met weekly for a two-hour prayer session.

The three groups had no contact or communication with each other. They were given several psychological tests before and after the experiment. All tests were administered by a skilled psychometrist with a degree in psychology, who was not directedly involved in the experiment. The tests included the Rorschach or "ink blot" test, which reveals something of the inner dynamics of the personality; the Szondi test, which gives further insight into certain personality syndromes; the Thematic Apperception test or TAT, which assesses through free expression a person's inner attitudes and feelings; and Sentence Completion and Word Association tests, which do much the same.

The results of these tests were made available to the counselors in the psychotherapy group, who used them to guide patients through therapy. The prayer therapy group (Group III) also made use of the test results. Each week each member received a sealed envelope containing a slip of paper on which was written a detrimental aspect of his or her personality that had been revealed on the tests. This allowed the person to focus on the negative trait and try to eliminate it by a specific prayer. As the prayer group continued to meet, the participants began to share the results of their tests, the barriers they encountered in dealing with them as well as their successes. The results of the tests were also known to the psychologist and his assistants who were running the overall experiment.

Nine months later the patients were given all the tests once again by an impartial psychologist. The results, as described by the researchers: Group I, the psychotherapy group, had a 65 percent improvement. Group II, the self-prayer, had no improvement. And Group III, the prayer therapy group, had a 72 percent improvement.

In their appraisal of these results, the researchers expressed delight with the outcome. They were convinced that they had witnessed "total healing" in several participants in Group III, the prayer therapy group, of conditions that included migraine headaches, stuttering, ulcers, and epilepsy. For them the power of prayer, when combined with information to the subjects about the results of their psychological testing, was evident.

On the surface it is difficult to understand the enthusiasm of the researchers over Group III's results. Even if the estimates of improvement are accurate, which is difficult to verify because no solid endpoints were being measured, the prayer therapy Group III did only 7 *percent* better than the prayerless Group I—a very meager achievement.

In addition there is no way to know what accounted for their improvement. At least three factors were at work: prayer, group therapy, and individual feedback about the results of their psychological tests. It is not possible to separate the effects of these variables. Any of these factors could have made all the difference, part of the difference, or no difference at all; we simply do not know.

Why would God answer prayers only for Group III? Why would it be necessary, for him to answer prayer, to have people gathered in a group, and to have them assisted with knowledge of the results of their psychological tests? One could argue that, rather than demonstrating the *power* of prayer, Group III's results demonstrate God's limitations or his capriciousness.

Why didn't Group II—Christians praying for themselves in privacy—improve? The explanation of the researchers was that "something was wrong with prayer as understood and practiced" by them. Since they "asked and received not," they must have somehow unknowingly "asked amiss," while the Group III participants "asked and received." This is unconvincing; for it ignores the fact that the prayerless Group I patients also "received," and did not even ask.

There is indication that the Group III participants felt that the group therapy factor was extremely important. All of them wished to come back the following year and continue the group.

Can we believe the data generated by this study? Are the percentages of improvements reliable? As almost everyone knows, psychological tests are at best general indicators of forces at work in the psyche; to use them to prove precise percentages of improvement is probably going too far. Accurate, empirical criteria for improvement of medical conditions are missing from this experiment. For example, one can only know if the reported ulcer actually healed by looking at it in some way—by using X rays or a fiberoptic gastroscope. Relying on symptoms is notoriously unreliable: some active ulcers are painless, while some patients have ulcer-type pain without having an actual ulcer.

These are the conclusions of the chief experimenter of the Redlands study:

> Repeatedly, under scientific test conditions, divorced from incense or high emotional persuasion, I have seen [the] beneficent results [of prayer]. . . . we have experimented with prayer under conditions satisfying all the demands of modern "scientific" man. . . . In nine months, for the first time in history, the results of a controlled experiment in prayer . . . [was] scientifically measured, compared, and evaluated.[7]

But this experiment, in my judgment, is not a convincing demonstration of the power of prayer. It is riddled with problems; it simply is not good science.

Childhood Leukemia and Prayer

Skeptics of prayer generally state that any proof that prayer is effective is due only to poorly designed experiments and observations and is therefore an illusion. If the experiments are airtight, the effect will be eliminated. Prayer violates the known laws governing physical reality; therefore we know in advance that it cannot work.

A study frequently cited by skeptics to prove these contentions is a prayer experiment performed on children with leukemia, reported in 1965.[8] A researcher randomly assigned ten of eighteen leukemic children for treatment by a prayer group at a church. All eighteen children continued their routine medical treatments. Ten families were asked to pray at the church for the ten children, and they received weekly reminders of their obligation to pray. Neither the children nor their treating physicians knew they were subjects of an experiment in prayer, nor did the praying families know that a controlled study was going on. The results of this study were inconclusive, with no significant differences between the two groups.

Skeptics of prayer seem generally elated about this outcome and seldom fail to cite it as proof against the effectiveness of prayer. But as Daniel J. Benor, M.D.,[9] has observed, "There are so many flaws in the study it is an embarrassment to anyone with research experience." In fact it is *so* flawed that it reflects poorly on skeptics, who claim to be scientists, to tout it as decisive proof against prayer. Some of the reasons this study was doomed from the start are as follows:

• There were too few patients on which to base conclusions.

• No assessment was given about the comparability of the two groups—that is, one cannot tell if one group was sicker than the other, which would have skewed the outcome.

• The patients did not even have the same illness. Two patients in the control (unprayed-for) group had myelogenous leukemia, whereas all other patients in both groups had lymphatic leukemia. This fact is crucial because leukemia is not a homogenous disease; some forms have a worse prognosis than others.

• No information is given as to the comparability of the two groups as to other important variables such as age and sex.

• Criteria for improvement are not specified.

• No checks were made to see whether families committed to prayer actually kept their obligation and if so, how often they prayed.

• Neither can we tell anything about the variability of chemo-therapy treatment in the children, which might have accounted for the variations in responses.

Like the Redlands experiment, this study's poor design renders its findings inconclusive.

Prayer and Rheumatoid Arthritis

Another well-known study that attempted to assess the possible power of prayer in patients with rheumatoid arthritis was re-ported in 1965 from a London hospital. This was a double-blind study: neither the patients nor physicians knew who was and who was not being prayed for. Distant prayer groups offered prayer to nineteen pa-tients, whose course was compared to that of nineteen control patients. Researchers matched the two groups as to the severity of their disease. Medical therapy was continued as usual in both the control and experi-mental groups. The patients were carefully evaluated at the beginning of the study and again after eight to eighteen months. Only six of the thirty-eight patients improved; five of these were in the prayer group. During the first half of the study, the prayer group improved more than did the control group; but in the last half of the study, the control group improved more. While these results are encouraging for an ef-fect of prayer, researchers found no statistical significance in this small study. Overall this experiment contributes little to our scientific under-standing of prayer.[10]

Prayer Involving Human Tissue

If our thoughts can affect "lower" biological systems, suggested in many of the studies that follow, some researchers have suggested that living, human tissue might be even more responsive to these effects. If so, what kind of human tissue would be most sensitive?

Nobel neurophysiologist Sir John Eccles has proposed that the human brain is exquisitely sensitive to thought. As he put it, the mind exerts continual "cognitive caresses" on the millions of neurons that make up the brain.[11] Might the brain's sensitivity to thought make it more likely to respond to not only our inner thoughts, but to the mental efforts of other persons such as healers, who might be at a distance?

It is difficult to use living brain tissue experimentally as a distant target for thought. We must obtain brain tissue surgically via biopsy, which involves risk. It is far easier to use other body tissue, such as various types of blood cells. Certain blood cells have a lot in common with brain tissue. For example, many white blood cells contain identical receptor sites for neurotransmitter molecules that exist also in the brain, and they manufacture some of these substances as well. So if mind "cognitively caresses" brain tissue, might it similarly affect blood cells that are functionally similar?

Dr. William G. Braud of the Mind Science Foundation in San Antonio, Texas, put this question to the test.[12] He wanted to know 1. whether or not ordinary people can mentally protect red blood cells from serious, stressful influences; 2. whether this could be done at a distance; and 3. whether this effect is "selfish"—that is, whether the mentally protective effect works better on a subject's own red blood cells, or whether it equally protects the cells of others.

In Braud's experiment thirty-two subjects—seventeen females and fifteen males, ranging in age from twenty-three to fifty-three years— mentally attempted to keep red blood cells (RBCs) from dissolving when they were placed in test tubes containing a dilute solution in a distant room. This is stressful for RBCs; they gradually swell and burst, leaking their hemoglobin into the solution. This process, known as hemolysis, can be measured with extreme accuracy with a device known as a spectrophotometer.

Approximately half of Braud's subjects were instructed to try mentally to protect their *own* blood cells, while half were assigned to protect blood cells of *another* person. It is important to note that the subjects were "blind"—that is, they did not know if the blood came from their own body or from someone else. During each session the subjects were placed in a quiet, comfortable room in one part of the building, and the target, the tubes of blood, was placed in a distant room in the same building. A session consisted of two control or rest periods of fifteen minutes each and two fifteen-minute "protect" periods. As an aid to visualization and intention, they looked at a color slide projection of healthy, intact RBCs. During the control periods, the subjects closed their eyes and thought about matters not connected with the experiment. The technician performing the hemolysis measurements on the RBCs in the distant room was also "blind"—ignorant as to whether the blood originated from the subject or someone else, and ignorant also as to whether a control or a "protect" session was in progress.

Braud reached two important conclusions. First, the subjects could influence the rate of hemolysis of the distant RBCs to a degree unexplainable by chance. Second, the source of the blood was not significant in the group *as a whole*. However, when *individual* performances were examined, the five most skillful subjects in the entire experiment were those trying to influence their own blood.

This study suggests that healing thoughts can function at a distance, and that they are *on the whole* unselfish. They seem to occur regardless of whether they are directed to one's self or to another. But although the *overall* effect seems unselfish when large groups of people are studied, there also appear to be individuals who are not typical of the entire group, people whose healing thoughts may be more potent for themselves than for others.

What makes the difference? Braud suggests that the mental strategies that each individual employs may be important. In his study some people used images in which the RBCs were visualized in a very realistic manner. Other people used mental images involving objects similar but not identical to the RBCs, but which possessed qualities that a strong, protected cell might possess. Braud also suggests that personality differences among subjects may affect the results. Some personality types might feel more comfortable with a highly specific and graphic form of imagery, some with an indirect or nonspecific mental strategy.

Prayer in the Coronary Care Unit

Cardiologist Randolph Byrd, a practicing Christian, designed his study as a scientific evaluation of the role of God in healing. "After much prayer," he states, "the idea of what to do came to me."[13] Over a ten-month period, a computer assigned 393 patients admitted to the coronary care unit at San Francisco General Hospital to

either a group that was prayed for by home prayer groups (192 patients) or to a group that was not remembered in prayer (201 patients).
The study was designed according to rigid criteria, the kind usually
used in clinical studies in medicine. It was a randomized, double-blind
experiment in which neither the patients, nurses, nor doctors knew
which group the patients were in. Byrd recruited various religious
groups to pray for members of the designated prayed-for group. The
prayer groups were given the first names of their patients as well as a
brief description of their diagnosis and condition. They were asked to
pray each day, but were given no instructions on how to pray. "Each
person prayed for many different patients, but each patient in the experiment had between five and seven people praying for him or her,"
Byrd explained.

The prayed-for patients differed in several areas:

1. They were five times less likely than the unremembered group
to require antibiotics (three patients compared to sixteen patients).

2. They were three times less likely to develop pulmonary edema,
a condition in which the lungs fill with fluid as a consequence of the
failure of the heart to pump properly (six compared to eighteen patients).

3. None of the prayed-for group required endotracheal intubation, in which an artificial airway is inserted in the throat and attached
to a mechanical ventilator, while twelve in the unremembered group
required mechanical ventilatory support.

4. Fewer patients in the prayed-for group died (although this difference was not statistically significant).

If the technique being studied had been a new drug or a surgical
procedure instead of prayer, it would almost certainly have been heralded as some sort of "breakthrough." Even some hardboiled skeptics
agreed on the significance of Byrd's findings. Dr. William Nolan, who
has written a book debunking faith healing, acknowledged, "It sounds
like this study will stand up to scrutiny. . . . maybe we doctors ought to
be writing on our order sheets, 'Pray three times a day.' If it works, it
works."[14]

When the results of Dr. Byrd's study were announced, they created a sensation. News of the experiment was carried on every major
wire service in the United States. Believers felt that at long last a careful

study had finally demonstrated a profound effect of prayer. The skeptics finally would be silenced and the scientific community convinced that prayer works. This was not to be. Since the study was published, it has come under sharp criticism. Some of the objections are as follows.

The Born-Again Factor

The study recruited only "born-again" Christians, who were to pray to their Christian God. They had "an active Christian life as manifested by daily devotional prayer and active Christian fellowship with a local church." Several Protestant churches and the Roman Catholic church were represented. Some critics of this study have wondered, in view of these selection criteria, whether Byrd may have had a religious ax to grind, a hidden agenda to prove the superiority of his personal religion.

Did Prayer Actually Occur?

The praying people—the intercessors—were instructed "to pray daily for a rapid recovery and for prevention of complications and death, in addition to other areas of prayer they believed to be beneficial to the patient." Yet there were no safeguards to determine if the prayer groups really prayed or not.

Prayer Strategies

The praying people or intercessors were told only to pray, not how to pray, and were not asked about the methods they employed. Thus we know little of the prayer strategies used. But as we've seen earlier, prayer is "not just" prayer. Many factors are involved in its outcome, including the degree of specificity or directedness of the prayer. For instance, the Spindrift researchers found that a *nondirected* form of prayer, in which no specific goal or outcome is attached (the "Thy will be done" attitude), was two to four times more effective than a directed method (see chapter 5). Other authorities have suggested that prayer methods should be tailored to one's personality if they are to be effective (see chapter 5). These factors went unexamined in the Byrd study. The meager outcome of this experiment may therefore reflect the way the study was designed rather than on the intrinsic effects of prayer.

The Skill Factor

Assessing the skills and experience of the praying people seems important in any prayer study, just as one would consider the skills of an internist or neurosurgeon to be crucial in any medical experiment. Evidence from the Spindrift studies suggests that some people are simply more effective than others when praying. Experience counts—about which we know nothing in Byrd's experiment.

Familiarity and Prayer

The Spindrift experiments also demonstrated that prayer is more effective if the praying person is familiar with the object of prayer. Although the intercessors in the Byrd experiment knew the first name, diagnosis, and a bit about the clinical condition of the patients they were praying for, they had no personal knowledge of the sick person, no familiarity in any meaningful sense. Judging from the Spindrift experiments, this could have diminished significantly the results that were observed.

The First-Name Factor

Because each patient in the prayer group was assigned to three to seven intercessors, who were given the patient's first name, diagnosis, and general condition, along with pertinent updates in their general condition, some skeptics have pointed out that this violates the double-blind design of the experiment. For the study to be genuinely double-blind, the intercessors should have been kept totally in the dark. Although this is technically a valid objection, this seems to be an extremely trivial criticism. If prayer really works, who would care if the praying person knew about the patient's condition?

Providing the intercessors with the first names of the patients creates a potentially interesting problem. Presumably there were several people with the same first names in the total 393 patients. What if there were Johns and Marys in *both* the control and prayer groups? If the intercessor prayed for "John" or "Mary," *which* John or Mary would receive the prayer? Could the prayer have been inadvertently directed to the Johns and Marys in the control group instead of the prayed-for group, as intended? Could the effect of prayer have "leaked" into the control group because of this confusion? Granted that God knows the difference, but why was this obvious factor not eliminated from the experimental design at the start, perhaps by eliminating all names and assigning numbers or initials to the patients? One is reminded of a comment by C. S. Lewis in his *Letters to Malcolm: Chiefly on Prayer*: ". . . [W]hy you find it so important to pray for people by their Christian names I can't imagine. I always assume God knows their surnames as well."[15]

Doctor Differences

We also know nothing about the skills of the various physicians caring for the patients. The expertise of physicians differs, of course, as does that of nurses and other members of the health care team. Some doctors are more prone to use medications than others; some are quicker to intubate patients and mechanically ventilate them; some keep their patients in the coronary care unit longer than others. Since all these factors were used in assessing the effects of prayer, some evaluation of the treatment habits of the doctors involved would have been desirable. If doctors who were less inclined to use diuretics and antibiotics cared predominantly for patients in the prayer group, the lower incidence of use of these drugs might have reflected *not* the effect of prayer, but the conservative prescribing habits of the physicians. Granted, this information would have been extremely tedious or even impossible to obtain, but this does not annul its importance.

Effects of Psychological Denial

There was no attempt to assess the psychological coping mechanisms of the patients in the coronary care unit (CCU). This may have been a crucial flaw in the experiment. Based on studies done at Harvard Medical School, we know that the most effective psychological coping strategy during the first twenty-four hours following a heart attack is *denial*. People who deny what is happening to them early in the CCU experience less anxiety, fewer cardiac arrhythmias, and a lower mortality.[16] If there were more deniers in the prayed-for group, this factor instead of intercessory prayer might have accounted for the improvements.

"Outside" Prayer

We do not know whether or how much the patients in the control group prayed for themselves, or whether their relatives prayed for them. Since we can presume that *some* of them prayed for themselves or were prayed for by relatives, this means that in effect there was *no* control group, no group *not* being prayed for. Since this factor was not assessed, for all we know the control group may have been prayed for *more* than the formal prayer group. If so, this would mean that the most-prayed-for group did worse—in which case the entire study might be interpreted as evidence not that prayer works, but that it is actually harmful.

Byrd acknowledges the difficulty in keeping track of the prayer involved. "[There was no] attempt to limit prayer among the controls," he says. "Such action would certainly be unethical and probably impossible to achieve," with which I agree.

Divine Power or Divine Limitation?

In spite of prayers for a rapid recovery, there was no difference between the two groups either in the total number of days in the hospital or the coronary care unit. Neither was there a difference in the number of discharge medications given to the patients in the two groups. There also was no statistical difference in mortality: thirteen prayed-for patients (7 percent) and seventeen control patients (8.5 percent) died. Even in areas where statistical significance was observed, the superiority of the prayer group was not overwhelming: only 7 percent fewer required antibiotics; 5 percent fewer required diuretics; and there were 5 percent fewer cases of pneumonia, 6 percent fewer instances of congestive heart failure, and 5 percent fewer instances of cardiopulmonary arrest.

Overall 85 percent of the prayer group were judged to have a "good hospital course" after entry, compared to 73 percent of the control group. The most impressive difference was the need for intubation and mechanical ventilation: none of the prayed-for patients required such, while twelve of the controls received this intervention. This means that, except for one category of clinical response, *the prayed-for patients achieved only a 5 to 7 percent improvement over the controls.* If prayer works, why these minimal differences? Some cynics have stated that these marginal improvements, if real, indicate not God's power but his weakness.

Dr. Gary P. Posner, an internist in Tampa, Florida, is skeptical of Byrd's results and has attacked them on several grounds. The patients in the control group, he says, were just as worthy of being healed as the prayed-for group, and for God to favor one group over the other is a blight on his omniscience and compassion.[17]

Are Prayer Experiments Ethical?

One might wonder how anyone who devoutly believes in the power of prayer in healing could engage in a stringently controlled human experiment in the first place. For such a believer, withholding prayer from the control group might seem equivalent to denying them treatment with a potent drug or surgical procedure, which appears unethical and immoral.

In spite of the difficulties and problems with his study, I believe Byrd is to be congratulated for his courage in executing such an experiment in a modern medical environment. Most medical researchers would have shrunk from the task. Performing prayer research is hardly the way to further one's career; it does little to insure promotion or tenure; it does not enhance one's stature among colleagues. And to his credit, Byrd is not evangelical about his results. He concludes only that these data "suggest" that intercessory prayer has an effect in patients admitted to the coronary care unit.

But what have we learned? Do we know any more about the possible effects of prayer as a result of this experiment? I am afraid the answer may be no. Admittedly the fact that no prayed-for patients required intubation and mechanically assisted breathing, compared to twelve in the nonprayer group, is *extremely* impressive. And while only four fewer patients died in the prayed-for group (thirteen compared to seventeen), if we were among the survivors we would really not care that this difference did not reach statistical significance. For us it would be *highly* significant to be alive: damn the statistics. On balance, however, one is tempted to believe that this study has missed the mark. The main reason: if prayer works, we would expect evidence greater than a few small percentage points of improvement. We would want to see statistically significant life-or-death effects, which simply did not occur.

When it comes to proof of the power of prayer, we want more than a seven-percentage-point advantage. We want more than a "suggestion" that prayer works.

Byrd's study could be improved in many ways, as implied above. But some of these seem hopelessly difficult to assess. For instance, it might be possible to insure that the intercessors prayed, but how could we ever know if they were sincere and really "meant it"? How can we judge their skills and past experience in praying? How can we monitor the different strategies used by all the intercessors? And what about the key variable of physician and nursing skills? These challenges are complex and are likely to confound any future study of prayer in human beings.

I feel the Byrd experiment is suggestive but inconclusive and inherently ambiguous. It simply contains too many problems that prevent us from drawing firm conclusions about the possible power of prayer. In fact *all* the human prayer studies we have examined so far fall into this category.

In view of these problems, many researchers feel it is easier to study the effects of prayer in simple, *nonhuman* living systems. Prayer experiments in simpler life forms are much less ambiguous, involve fewer variables, and are easier to interpret. That is why they are so important.

Effects on Human Beings

In another study done at the Mind Science Foundation in San Antonio, Texas, researchers William G. Braud and Marilyn Schlitz studied the ability of sixty-two people to influence the physiology of 271 subjects. The subjects were isolated from the influencers, in distant rooms in the same building. Participants ranged from sixteen to sixty-five years, and were selected from a pool of volunteers from the San Antonio community. They had learned about the experiments through local newspaper ads and articles, notices, lectures given by the Foundation staff, and through comments by other participants. Approximately equal numbers of males and females were involved.

Thirteen experiments were done. The subjects were not selected on the basis of any special physical, physiological, or psychological characteristics, only their interest in the research. Only in one experiment were "special" subjects recruited—those in need of a "calming" influence on their physiology. That is, these subjects had evidence of greater than usual sympathetic autonomic activation as evidenced by stress-related complaints, excessive emotionality, excessive activity, tension headaches, high blood pressure, ulcers, or mental or physical hyperactivity. Prior to the experiment, they were screened by tests confirming that they did indeed exhibit greater than average arousal of the sympathetic nervous system.

The subjects, whose physiology the influencers were attempting to change, were attached to sensitive instruments measuring their electrodermal activity—the ability of the skin to conduct an electrical current, which is an indicator of activity of the sympathetic part of the autonomic nervous system. At a given signal, the influencer would try to exert a *calming* or an *activation* of the distant subject, who was unaware when the attempt would be made. In each session the influencer made twenty thirty-second attempts. During these "influence periods," the influencer used mental imagery and self-regulation techniques in order to induce the intended condition (either relaxation or activation, as demanded by the experimental protocol) in *himself* or *herself*, and imagined and intended a corresponding change in the distant subject. Then the influencer would imagine the desired outcomes of the polygraph pen tracings—a few small pen deflections for calming periods, and many large pen deflections for activation periods.

The intentions seemed to "get through" to the subjects. The effect proved to be consistent, replicable, and robust. "Under certain conditions," the researchers noted, "the transpersonal imagery effect can compare favorably with an imagery effect upon one's own physiological activity."

In some of the experiments, it seemed that specific images were being transmitted from influencer to subject. For example, a subject reported spontaneously that during the session he had a very vivid impression of the influencer coming into his room, walking behind his chair, and vigorously shaking the chair; the impression was so strong that he found it difficult to believe that the event had not happened in reality. This session was one in which the influencer had employed just such an image in order to activate the subject from afar.

At the beginning of one session, the experimenter remarked to an influencer that the electrodermal tracings of the subject were very precise and regimented and that they reminded him of the German techno-pop instrumental musical group Kraftwerk. When the experimenter went to the subject's room at the end of the session, the subject's first comment was that early in the session, for some unknown reason, thoughts of the group Kraftwerk had come into her mind. The subject could not have overheard the experimenter's earlier comment. "Such correspondences were not rare."

These thirteen experiments, involving a total of 333 influencers and subjects, contain certain lessons:

• The transpersonal imagery effect compares favorably with the magnitude of one's individual thoughts, feelings, and emotions on one's own physiology.

• This ability is apparently widespread in the population.

• It can occur at distances of twenty meters (greater distances were not tested).

• Subjects with a greater need to be influenced—that is, those for whom the influence would be beneficial—seem more susceptible.

• This effect can occur without the subject's knowledge.

• Those participating in these studies seemed unconcerned that the effect would be used for harm, and there is no evidence that harm occurred.

• The transpersonal imagery effect is not invariable. Subjects appear capable of shielding or preventing the effect if it is unwanted.

• The researchers suspect that certain psychological conditions in the subject, the influencer, or the *experimenter* may play a role in the success of the imagery. Factors such as confidence, belief, positive expectation, motivation, level of spontaneity, mood, and rapport may be among the factors affecting success of the imagery attempts.

What is the relation between transpersonal imagery and prayer? Both prayer and imagery have in common the ability to bring about helpful changes in the bodies of others at a distance, without the subject's conscious awareness. If God is included in the "loop," does this increase the overall effect, making prayer more effective than godless imagery? Or does God appear content to work through imagery and visualization without being explicitly acknowledged in the process?

These questions have not been answered by any of the research we've looked at.

THE NONHUMAN STUDIES

As an example of the apprehension that exists in medical institutions about spiritual healing, consider a true story that originated in a large hospital. Several nurses became interested in learning Therapeutic Touch, a technique developed by nurse-academician Dolores Krieger of New York University. This technique, a variation of the ancient practice of laying-on of hands, has been scientifically studied in several carefully controlled experiments. One weekend these nurses went away to take a course in this technique, which apparently infuriated the director of nursing. When the nurses returned to work on Monday morning, fresh from the course, they were met by a large sign on the bulletin board in the nursing department: THERE WILL BE NO HEALING IN THIS HOSPITAL!

One of the best-kept secrets in medical science is the extensive experimental evidence for "spiritual healing." Daniel J. Benor, M.D., an American psychiatrist working in England, surveyed all such healing studies published in the English language prior to 1990. He defined "spiritual healing" as "the intentional influence of one or more people upon another living system without utilising known physical means of intervention." His search turned up 131 studies, most of them in nonhumans. In fifty-six of these studies, there was less than one chance in a hundred that the positive results were due to chance. In an additional twenty-one studies, the possibility of a chance explanation was between two and five chances in a hundred.[18]

Why is this information relatively unknown? Medical journals have generally refused, until recently, to publish studies on healing. One of Benor's reasons for performing this exhaustive review was to bring together in one place this body of research so it could be easily surveyed by the medical community. The actual citations of these studies can be found in Appendix 1. We cannot examine all of them, and will therefore select only a few of the fifty-six that yielded significant results. I hope these examples will convey the nature of the research done in this area.

Effects on Fungi, Yeast, and Bacteria

A number of studies have researched the effects of healing on fungi, yeast, or bacteria. The following are some of the results.

• Ten subjects tried to inhibit the growth of fungus cultures in the laboratory through conscious intent by concentrating on them for fifteen minutes from a distance of approximately 1.5 yards. The cultures were then incubated for several more hours. Of a total of 194 culture dishes, 151 showed retarded growth.[19]

• In a replication of this study, one group of subjects demonstrated the same effect (inhibiting the growth of the fungus) in sixteen out of sixteen trials, while stationed from one to fifteen *miles* away from the fungus cultures.[20]

• Sixty subjects not known to have healing abilities were able both to impede *and* stimulate significantly the growth of cultures of bacteria.[21]

• In a similar experiment, two healers held a bottle of water in their hands for thirty minutes. Samples of the water were then added to solutions of yeast cells in test tubes. After incubation the amount of carbon dioxide given off by the yeast cultures was measured, indicating the level of metabolic activity. Statistically significant increases in carbon dioxide production were observed by the yeast cultures given the "treated" water in four of five tests.[22]

• Sixty university volunteers with no known healing abilities were asked to alter the genetic ability of a strain of the bacteria *Escherichia coli*, which normally mutates from the inability to metabolize the sugar lactose ("lactose negative") to the ability to use it ("lactose positive") at a known rate. The subjects tried to influence nine test tubes of bacterial cultures—three for increased mutation from lactose negative to lactose positive, three for decreased mutation of lactose negative to lactose positive, and three tubes uninfluenced as controls. Results indicated that the bacteria indeed mutated in the directions desired by the subjects.[23]

These experiments have implications for health and illness. Among them:

1. There may be times when it would be helpful to inhibit the growth of pathogenic microorganisms, as in the case of infections. On the other hand, our bodies contain helpful, symbiotic microorganisms whose growth might need to be increased on certain occasions, such as after treatment with antibiotics, which kill "good" bacteria in addition to pathogenic ones. The ability to inhibit or increase the growth of bacterial or yeast populations could be a valuable health resource.

2. If genetic mutations can be influenced by the conscious efforts of others, as in one of the above studies, then genes cannot be the absolute controllers they are represented to be. Biology, therefore, is not destiny.

For most people, "mutation" has negative connotations, as when a normal gene mutates to a cancerous one. Recent evidence shows the reverse can happen: abnormal genes can mutate to normal ones. This phenomenon, called "reverse mutation," has been discovered to occur in myotonic dystrophy, a disease causing severe muscle weakness and which strikes one in eighty thousand people.[24] Scientists don't know what causes "good" mutations. Could the mind be involved? The above evidence suggests that we should not rule out the possibility.

3. Many believers in spiritual healing claim that for healing to occur subjects must actively want it. These studies suggest otherwise. We can assume that the microorganisms did not know they were subjects in an experiment. The observed effects do not depend on what the subject thinks.

4. These experiments support the universal claim of healers that spiritual healing operates as powerfully at a distance as it does nearby.

5. Based on these studies, it seems that ordinary people have the ability to bring about biological changes in other living organisms. This suggests that everyone may possess innate healing abilities, at least to some degree.

6. Negative effects (inhibition of growth) as well as positive effects (promotion of growth) were observed in the above experiments. This raises the possibility of a dark side to healing, already examined in chapter 9.

7. Although skeptics often criticize spiritual healing as being simply the result of suggestion or a placebo response, the above experiments

show that this cannot be true, unless skeptics wish to attribute a high degree of consciousness to bacteria and yeast. These results suggest that the effects of spiritual healing can be completely independent of the "psychology" of the subject.

Effects on Cells

Cancer cells normally stick to the surface of the container in which they are being cultured. Changes in their metabolism, injury, or death cause them to detach and slough off into the surrounding medium. Researchers can count the number of cells in the medium and thus judge the overall state of health of the cell culture.

British psychic Matthew Manning held his hands near flasks containing cancer cells and attempted to inhibit their growth. He was able to produce changes of 200 percent to 1,200 percent in their growth characteristics when they were assessed as described. He influenced them even when he was placed in a distant room that was shielded from electrical influences.[25]

Effects on the Movement of Simple Organisms

Several experiments have examined the ability of subjects to affect not the growth but the movement of simple organisms. The motility and speed of motion of one-celled algae and paramecia, and the movement characteristics of moth larvae, have been significantly affected intentionally in a variety of experiments.[26]

Effects on Plants

In a well-known series of experiments, Dr. Bernard Grad of McGill University studied the healer Oskar Estebany, who claimed he could transmit his healing through paper, water, and other materials. Grad damaged barley seeds by watering them with a 1 percent saline solution, which retards their normal growth rate. He found that the damaging effect of the saline could be inhibited if Estebany held the container of saline for fifteen minutes.[27]

As Benor notes, "The administration of healing via secondary materials [here, the saline] which appears to carry the healing effect has been reported since Biblical times. It would appear . . . that there may be substance to these claims." But if spiritual healing is possible, as these many experiments suggest, why wouldn't the healer deal directly with the subject? Why use secondary materials as a "go between"? The reason may have to do with the personality of the healer. Psychologist LeShan has proposed that some healers don't feel comfortable "becoming one" with the subject. Using a secondary material such as water may allow them to distance themselves in the healing process.

Healing Effects on Animals

Many studies have been performed to determine the effects of healing methods on animals. Some of the results are detailed below.

• In an oft-quoted classic study, Grad studied Estebany's ability to heal artificially created surgical wounds in forty-eight mice, compared to a control group who were wounded identically (the wounds were created by removing a 1/2 × 1-inch piece of skin from their backs after anesthetizing them). Estebany held the cages of the experimental group fifteen minutes twice daily for fourteen days. This group healed significantly faster than the wounded mice whose cages were not held. This careful study once again tells us that healing works and that it is not just due to suggestion.[28]

• In another experiment Grad produced goiters in mice by giving them a diet devoid of iodine in addition to thiouracil, a goiter-producing drug. Estebany held the cages of one group of rats for fifteen minutes twice daily. This seemed to protect their thyroid glands from enlarging. Compared to a control group, the glands of the treatment group grew significantly slower than the controls.[29]

• In a subsequent experiment, Grad tested Estebany's claim that healing effects could be transmitted by secondary materials. In an experiment similar to the above, Estebany held some wool or cotton in his hands, which was then placed in the rats' cages for one hour, morning and evening, six days a week. The thyroid glands of the rats receiving this treatment grew significantly more slowly than the controls; and when the rats were returned to an iodine-containing diet, they returned to normal size more quickly than controls.[30]

• In twenty-one experiments conducted over a period of several years, healers tried to awaken mice more quickly from general anesthesia. These experiments were increasingly refined. In one variation only the image of the experimental mouse was projected on a TV monitor to the healer in a distant room, who tried to intervene via the image. Nineteen of the twenty-one studies showed highly significant results: earlier recovery from anesthesia of the "treated" mice. The experimenters were able to identify a peculiar "linger effect" in this series of studies. They found that if one side of a table was used by the healers in recovering their mice, and that if the healers were then dismissed and more anesthetized rats were placed immediately on that side of the table, they recovered faster than controls placed on the table's other side.[31]

• In another experiment a group of mice were injected with either a strain of malaria organisms or with sterile saline. The handlers of the mice were told that the injection contained either a "high dose" or "low dose" of microorganisms. They also were informed that a healer would try to heal some of the rats but not others. In fact the handlers were deceived: *there was no high or low dose* (the malaria injections were identical); and *no healer was employed*. In one phase of the experiment, the results tended in the direction of the expectations of the handlers: the rats *believed* to have had high-dose injections did worse, and those *believed* to have had the low-dose injections did better. In addition the mice coded for healing did better than those not designated to be healed, even though the information designating which groups were to be healed was unknown to the handlers. There should have been no differences between the high-dose and low-dose groups, since there was no difference in the strength of the injections; and there should have been no difference between the healed and nonhealed groups, since there was no healer.[32]

This experiment raises profound questions about whether the double-blind experimental design used in medical research is as foolproof as believed. In double-blind situations, neither the experimenters nor the subjects know who is and is not receiving the treatment being studied, such as a new drug. Since the subjects don't know if they are receiving the drug or a placebo, they won't be as susceptible to the effects of suggestion; and since the experimenters are unaware which subjects received the drug and which did not, they will be less prone to bias when assessing any effects they observe in the subjects. We assume that these precautions eliminate the effects of expectation and suggestion in both the researchers and subjects. In the above study with malarial mice, however, the double-blind precautions were not sufficient: the outcome of the experiment mirrored the beliefs and expectations of the lab workers.

Similar findings have been seen in double-blind studies involving humans, as we saw in chapter 8. It appears that double-blind studies can sometimes be steered in directions that correspond to the thoughts and attitudes of the experimenters. This might shed light on why skeptical experimenters appear unable to replicate the findings of believers, and why "true believers" seem more able to produce positive results. The validity of decades of experimental findings in medical research would need to be reevaluated if it is proved that the mind can "shove the data around."

Chapter 12

What Is Healing?

> Pythagoras said that the most divine art was that of heal-
> ing. And if the healing art is most divine, it must occupy
> itself with the soul as well as with the body; for no crea-
> ture can be sound so long as the higher part in it is sickly.
>
> —Apollonius of Tyana

How does healing happen? Almost always in the stud-
ies we looked at in chapter 11, the healer employed a prayerful attitude,
if not actual prayer. This is one reason why many healers use the terms
"spiritual healing" and "prayer healing" interchangeably. Healers also
frequently use the term "centering" to describe this experiential state.
Centering requires the exclusion of extraneous, distracting thoughts
and feelings, focusing the attention on the immovable, central core of
being.[1]

Thus practically all types of spiritual healing make use of a
prayerful, meditative state of awareness. During this process the healer
adopts a dispassionate, loving, and compassionate attitude toward the
person in need. Psychologist Lawrence LeShan, who has studied spiritual healers extensively, describes this attitude as a feeling of selfless-
ness, a way of *being* instead of *doing:*

One can only be fully in this mode when one has, if only for a moment, given up all wishes and desires for oneself (since the separate self does not exist) and for others (since they do not exist as separate either) and just allow oneself to be and therefore to be with and be one with the all of existence . . . Any awareness of doing or of the wish to do disrupts this mode.[2]

This forgetting or going beyond the individual self—feeling united with each other and with the All—is frequently described by the healers studied by LeShan. Another crucial component common to their efforts is an immense caring and empathy for the person needing healing.[3] During this state the healer most often does not consider himself or herself to be the source of the healing, but only a conduit through which the healing flows from a higher power.

Distance, Time, and Energy

Although some of the studies surveyed by Benor involved healers who were only a few inches from the subject, some involved distances up to fifteen miles. Researcher William G. Braud says, "The 'operating characteristics' of the remote influence are . . . not . . . a function of spatial distance or time, and it is not influenced importantly by physical barriers, shields, or the nature of the particular system that is 'targeted.'"[4]

This means that none of the experiments reviewed so far can be explained by known physiological mechanisms, which localize conscious awareness and the effects of the mind to brains and bodies of individual people.

We simply don't know how the mind of one person can engage in "action at a distance" to bring about healthful changes in someone else. Yet healers continually speak as if they know. They most frequently describe their activities in the language of classical physics, saying that healing "energy" is "sent." But conventional forms of energy are an insufficient explanation for what we observe in spiritual healing experiments. In them the "energy" does not fade away with increasing distance, and it cannot be shielded, as we would expect if ordinary forms of energy were involved.

Perhaps, Braud states, the only conventional energy that may qualify as a potential mediator for distant healing is extremely low frequency (ELF) electromagnetic radiation. ELF is known to have excellent "penetrating" properties and little attenuation with distance. Some experimenters, such as Michael A. Persinger, have seriously proposed ELF fields as mediators for events like those we've discussed.[5] There are problems with that idea, Braud suggests. First, "[ELF fields] would have to behave in highly unusual ways with respect to *time* in order to explain the time-displaced mental effects that have been observed in certain experiments." (For example, in the Jahn-Dunne experiments, the receiver "gets" a complex mental image from the sender up to three days *before* it is selected by a computer and "sent" by the sender.) Second, ELF fields "would have to carry more information than they would appear capable of carrying." Third, "They would have to be encoded by the influencer's brain (or other bodily processes) and be decoded by the subject's brain (or other bodily processes) in ways that we do not understand and for which we have no known mechanisms. Therefore, an ELF-mediated carrier [as an explanation for distant healing effects] remains, while not entirely impossible, a highly implausible hypothesis."[6]

Robert G. Jahn and Brenda J. Dunne, the Princeton researchers whose experiments we have already examined, have freely acknowledged our ignorance about how consciousness interacts with the physical world. This includes our lack of understanding of prayer-based, spiritual healing and how one person can mentally affect the body of a distant individual. They state,

> The literature of psychic research abounds with attempts to transpose various physical formalisms [to account for these effects]: electromagnetic models, thermodynamic models, mechanical models, statistical mechanical models, hyperspace models, quantum mechanical models, and others. . . . Although these comprise an interesting body of effort, none of them seems fully competent. . . . Indeed, it appears that no simple application of existing physical theory is likely to prevail. In order to encompass the observed effects, a substantially more fundamental level of theoretical model will need be deployed, one which more explicitly acknowledges the role of consciousness in the definition of physical reality.[7]

We do not know how spiritual healing works, whether at close range or at a distance. Many skeptics argue that this is sufficient reason for tossing it out the window, completely rejecting it even as a possibility. But in view of the evidence favoring spiritual healing, this is a naive and reckless position.

To acknowledge that we don't know how something works is not a particularly damaging confession in medicine. No one knew how penicillin worked (or that it even existed) when Fleming made his famous observation that the growth of bacteria was inhibited by fungi. If the scientific community had used ignorance of the process as a justification for rejecting his discovery, the introduction of life-saving antibiotics would have been delayed. Similar examples abound. For centuries colchicine was known to be miraculously effective in relieving the pain of gout, one of the most intense forms of suffering known to humans. No one had a clue about its method of action until the modern era. The same holds true for the ability of aspirin to relieve pain and inflammation. The first question anyone suffering from infection, gout, or inflammation asks of any new therapy is not "*How* does it work?" but "*Does* it work?" As history shows, full explanations frequently come later. So it may be with prayer and spiritual healing.

WHY DO SCIENTISTS REJECT PRAYER-BASED HEALING?

Scientific evidence supporting spiritual healing is considerable. In addition to the 131 controlled experiments on prayer-based, "spiritual," "psychic," or "psi" healing reviewed by Benor, over half of which showed statistically significant results, psychologist William G. Braud reviewed 149 experiments with living "targets"—humans, mammals, or fish, for example—in which apparent telepathic influences affected their behavior in various ways.[8] Braud, like Benor, found that approximately half of these studies were statistically significant. Although the experiments reviewed by Braud do not deal with healing per use, they contribute significantly to the premise that mental efforts can affect living organisms at a distance, as in healing. Why are these findings—almost three hundred studies, dating back to the early 1960s—ignored or rejected by most scientists?

I believe the answer has less to do with the quality of the data than with the psychology of scientists themselves. I agree with Benor's hypothesis that "many critics would cloud the evidence with any excuses to support their disbeliefs rather than examine either the phenomena or their own discomforts with them." Benor is probably qualified to make such a claim; in addition to being a researcher in the field of spiritual healing, he is a trained psychiatrist as well.

Benor suggests various reasons why scientists and skeptics reject scientific evidence for distant healing.[9] Among them:

1. *Western materialistic beliefs exclude the possibility of prayer-based healing.* Because our modern scientific paradigm, or worldview, has no place for healing at a distance, it can be more convenient to ignore than engage the evidence for spiritual healing—the "if-it-can't-occur-it-doesn't-occur" approach. Modern medical science has become synonymous with the material, evidenced by our near-total reliance on drugs, surgery, radiation, and so on. The possibility that nonmaterial forms of healing might exist is virtually unthinkable.

2. *It is human nature to resist change.* It is emotionally comforting to believe that our views about the workings of the world are correct. When evidence to the contrary confronts us, it is natural to resist it.

3. *Cognitive dissonance* is a psychological term describing the discomfort people feel when there is a conflict between their perceptions and their belief system. Looking at evidence for distant healing stimulates this inner tension in some scientists. One way to resolve this discomfort is to derogate and reject the healing event without proper attention to evidence.

4. *Spiritual healing is often equated with "mysticism."* According to psychoanalytic theory, as children we struggle to differentiate between the inner worlds of the mind and the outer "physical" world, and then try to integrate the two. In our culture this almost always means attributing greater status to the outer than the inner world. Many intellectually oriented people, including scientists, seem to fear getting lost in the inner void of the mystic, which they unconsciously equate with emptiness, nothingness, annihilation, and death. The mystic, in contrast,

senses the void as the Source or *plenum*. As it is said, "The mystic swims in the sea in which the unmystical drown."

5. *Prayer-type healing may occur outside of conscious control.* This can be unsettling or frightening to someone who needs to be in conscious control most of the time, and who may inherently fear the workings of the unconscious.

6. *The "power of others" may be feared.* If someone can benevolently use their "power of the mind" at a distance, they might possibly use it in a negative way as well. This could expose one to the unseen influences of countless others, which can be fearful to contemplate.

7. *One's own healing powers may be feared.* If distant influences can operate at an unconscious level, what mischief might I be capable of without knowing it? It can be easier to deny that healing abilities exist than to take responsibility for using them.

8. *Healing power is believed to be possessed only by people who are strange or different.* People who are uncomfortable with healing may attribute these powers to mediums, guides, channelers, kooks, weirdos, or religious nuts. They may deny that average individuals, including themselves, possess these gifts. This permits them to dismiss those scientific studies that show that unskilled, ordinary people have inherent healing abilities.

In a variation of this defense, when they confront scientific evidence that healing can be done by ordinary individuals, they may erect unreasonably strict criteria in order to prove to themselves that healing is, after all, impossible for average folk. For instance, they may insist that healers perform on demand and on cue, under intense public scrutiny or actual distraction, and in sterile surroundings. By such tactics, Benor states, "they [assure] themselves that they will be unlikely to encounter an event which might upset them."

9. *The lack of replicability of healing phenomena* and their irregular occurrence in clinical settings is often used as justification to reject scientific studies out of hand. It is true that healers have not been able to produce results with reliability and consistency. The same healer might succeed a number of times but fail miserably in the next few trials. Researchers have not isolated the critical variables which can explain, much less predict, when healing will or won't happen. "Thus," observes Benor, "the physical scientists claim that healing phenomena are proba-

bly due to chance variations in the disease, 'spontaneous remissions' or other, unaccounted factors rather than results of healers' interventions."

This neglects the obvious: the nearly three hundred studies discussed above, over half of which show that people *can* exert healing influences on distant organisms at a statistically significant level. Some of these studies *have* been replicated.

We must consider "unpredictability" in context. Science accepts many phenomena that are inherently unpredictable, from electrons to earthquakes. The fact that it is now snowing outside my window, and that the weather bureau did not predict it, does not mean that it isn't happening. Neither does the fact that healers cannot perform predictably or on cue mean that they cannot heal.

What accounts for the unpredictability? "My guess," Benor offers, "is that shifting factors of boredom, beliefs and needs of participants shape the results into these observed patterns, along with numerous external factors."

10. *Healing has laws that appear to differ from those of other sciences.* Scientists insist that all phenomena obey the same laws, and that they consequently should be expected to jump through the same hoops experimentally. But this amounts to making "procrustean demands on researchers of healing," Benor says. "It is ludicrous that scientists from other fields should suggest that their rules for evidence should be applied in healing. . . . It would certainly be nicer, neater and less complicated if this worked. The fact that it does not work does not mean that healing does not exist."

Some researchers in healing have tried nonetheless to meet these expectations. For instance, some have tried to identify and provide a "standard dose" of healing that could be delivered by a healer across a uniform length of time. The assumption is that healing should work like drugs or irradiation, which are given in standard doses. Although some of these attempts have yielded positive results, the healers themselves reject this approach. They recognize that the length of time required to heal varies drastically between patients, but cannot say why. I agree with Benor, who believes we must recognize these limitations for what they are. "The time has come to accept that healing is the way it is," he asserts.

It appears to be influenced by multiple factors—so many, in fact, that it is virtually impossible to establish a repeatable experiment in which all would occur in the same combination more than once. As it is difficult to control any one of these, much less all of them in concert, it is little wonder that only approximately equivalent results have been obtained in experiments over numbers of trials. We will have to be content with our human limitations and settle for approximate results, measured in probabilities over large numbers of trials. No apologies are needed. These are the limitations of healing.

11. *Healing is often allied with specific religions that emphasize faith and belief.* C.S. Lewis once said, "The great religions were first preached and long practiced in a world without chloroform."[10] This implies that pain, suffering, and religious fervor go hand in hand. But now that science has arrived and transformed medicine, there is no real reason for medicine and religion to mix. Emphasizing the role of faith and belief in healing appears to be a step back in history for most scientists, and a justification for rejecting prayer-based healing.

12. *Careers and financial investments are at stake.* Almost all research grants, professorships, and health products are aligned with the physically based view of reality. It is small wonder that scientists involved in these activities do not automatically embrace experiments that call these assumptions into question.

The following apocryphal story illustrates the futility of further debate over many of these issues. A psychiatrist is treating a paranoid person who insists that he is dead. Having exhausted all ordinary arguments, the psychiatrist asks whether the patient knows that dead men don't bleed. He readily agrees they do not, and assents to have the psychiatrist prick his finger with a needle, which draws blood. "See, you're alive!" the psychiatrist declares triumphantly. "Wrong!" shouts the patient. "Dead men *do* bleed!"

Benor, who relates this tale, suggests that "those who feel the rightness of healing do not spend a lot of time arguing with those who do not, but rather get on with giving, receiving, and/or studying healing."

I am, on the whole, less pessimistic. Skeptics *do* change their minds occasionally when faced with evidence, and they especially modify their positions when they experience paranormal events personally, which is not uncommon.

And after all, it is a historical fact that science marches forward, frequently in spite of what most scientists think. As physicist Max Planck, whose discoveries launched the transition from classical to modern physics, put it: science changes, funeral by funeral.

PRAYER AND HEALING: WHAT LIES AHEAD?

Based on our observations, I'd like to make certain predictions for the future:

• The experimental evidence that nonlocal events permeate human experience will continue to accumulate. This will include the various ways in which consciousness acts at a distance, including through prayer.

• As physicians become increasingly comfortable with nonlocality as a legitimate concept in science, they will begin to use nonlocal interventions purposefully in both diagnosis and therapy. This will open the door widely to an Era III "nonlocal medicine" and will change the face of the profession. Nonlocal medicine will reject neither technological, mechanistic, Era I–type approaches, nor mind-body, Era II–type therapies, but will subsume them. The result will be a medicine that is both more effective and more humane, a medicine that works better and *feels* better.

• As nonlocal concepts find a home in medical science, prayer will become recognized as a potent force in medicine and will become incorporated into the mainstream.

• The use of prayer will become the standard in scientific medical practice in most medical communities.

• So pervasive will its use become that *not* to recommend the use of prayer as an integral part of medical care will one day constitute medical malpractice.

• The nonlocal nature of consciousness will be acknowledged in mainstream science because of conclusive evidence affirming it. It will become increasingly recognized that consciousness can do things the brain cannot.

• Having legitimized scientifically the existence of the nonlocal nature of consciousness, scientists and physicians will become more open to allowing nonlocality to manifest in their own lives. These "subjective proofs" will affirm and correlate with the objective, scientific studies that demonstrate that consciousness is nonlocal.

• A new picture of human consciousness will emerge. No longer will it be considered an exclusive byproduct of the brain, destined to die with the body.

• The recognition that there is some aspect of the human psyche that is genuinely nonlocal will lead to a transformation of our ideas of who we are. We will see that this nonlocal aspect of ourselves cannot die—for, if nonlocal, it is infinite in space and time, and thus omnipresent and immortal by implication.

• This soul-like quality of human beings will no longer be just an assertion of religions, to be accepted only through blind faith; it will be considered a legitimate implication of rational, empirical science.

• The recognition of a soul-like quality of consciousness—by science on the one hand and by religion on the other—will constitute a bridge between these two domains. This point of contact will help heal the bitter divisions between these two camps. No longer will people feel compelled to choose between them in ordering their lives. At long last science and religion will stand side by side in a complementary way, neither attempting to usurp the other.

• With the recognition that there is an innately nonlocal part of us that cannot die, the goals of medicine will be transformed. We shall come to realize that our intrinsic nonlocality constitutes an ever-present, Radical Cure—immortality—for the Big Disease, physical death.

• This recognition will not prohibit us from trying to eradicate illness, increase longevity, and prolong life; we may continue to do so if we so choose. But if so we shall no longer be acting out of desperation and fear of ultimate destruction at the moment of death. Rather we shall do so out of wisdom, recalling always that the most essential part of us cannot die, even in principle.

• This understanding may lead to a transformation in the way we pray. No longer will we pray incessantly *for things*, such as our health, but our prayers will be predominantly prayers of *gratitude* and *thanksgiving*—our proper response on realizing that the world, at heart, is more glorious, benevolent, and friendlier than we have recently supposed.

Afterword

A patient of mine was dying from lung cancer. The day before his death, I sat at his bedside with his wife and children. He knew he had little time left and he chose his words carefully, speaking in a hoarse whisper. Although not a religious person, he revealed to us that recently he had begun to pray frequently.

"What do you pray for?" I asked.

"I don't pray for anything," he responded. "How would I know what to ask for?" This was surprising. Surely this dying man could think of *some* request.

"If prayer is not for asking, what is it *for?*" I pushed him.

"It isn't 'for' anything," he said thoughtfully. "It mainly reminds me I am not alone."

Jiddu Krishnamurti, one of the most revered spiritual teachers of this century, once asked a small group of listeners what they would say to a close friend who is about to die. Their answers dealt with assurances, words about beginnings and endings, and various gestures of compassion. Krishnamurti stopped them short. There is only one thing you can say to give the deepest comfort, he said. Tell him that in his death a part of you dies and goes with him. Wherever he goes, you go also. He will not be alone.[1]

Prayer is like that. It is our tie to the Absolute, a reminder of our nonlocal, unbounded nature, of that part of us that is infinite in space and time and is Divine. It is the Universe's affirmation that we are immortal and eternal, that we are not alone.

We do not know why prayer reveals itself in scientific experiments, but we have seen that it does. What if it did not? Would it be less real?

In spite of its reputation as the most powerful arbiter of reality, it is nowhere written down that science is the only or the best gateway to what is real. We *invented* the scientific method; it did not descend from on high. Even if science's verdict on prayer were completely negative, that would not necessarily be the end of the story. And let us not deceive ourselves: Although science has much to say about prayer, it raises more questions than it answers. The mysteries of prayer not only remain, they deepen.

As we play the science-and-prayer game, as we have done in this book, let us always recall that it is *only* a game, a form of play. If play is to be genuine, it must be lighthearted and pursued without purpose. That is why we usually fail if we *try* to have fun. And that is also one reason that trying to "prove prayer" can be unsatisfying, in spite of the positive outcome of so many controlled experiments. Ultimately statistics don't satisfy, numbers don't nourish. So in spite of science's positive revelations about prayer, we continue to look beyond the laboratory to affirm the importance and meaning of prayer in our lives.

When we pray for the resolution of pain and suffering or any of the countless ways life tests us, and the prayer is not answered, it is not comforting to be reminded of prayer's "statistical significance" in a hundred laboratory experiments. At such moments it is only *our* "experiment" that counts. Why, we may lament, is the effect of prayer not more predictable, powerful, dependable? We need to recall at these times that prayer, in its function as a bridge to the Absolute, *has no failure rate*. It works 100 percent of the time—unless we prevent this realization by remaining oblivious to it.

We may wonder why prayer is so paradoxical and unpredictable, but the most astonishing fact is simply that it works at all—and not only in ways that can be tested in laboratory experiments, but in the most glorious and benevolent way imaginable—as a reminder of our origin and destiny: the Absolute, the Universal, the Divine.

Controlled Experimental
Trials of Healing

The following tables are the result of a survey by Daniel J. Benor, M.D., of studies on spiritual healing published in the English language. Originally appearing in the journal *Complementary Medical Research* in 1990, they will be expanded and updated in Benor's 1993 book, *Healing Research.* *

Benor defined healing as the *intentional influence of one or more people upon another living system without utilizing known physical means of intervention.* His findings:

- Researchers have performed 131 controlled trials.

- Fifty-six of these show statistically significant results at a probability level of <.01 or better (that is, the likelihood that the results were due to chance was less than 1 in 100).

- Twenty-one studies demonstrate results at a probability level of .02 to .05 (that is, the likelihood that the results were due to chance was between 2 and 5 chances in 100).

- These experiments deal with healing effects on enzymes, cells, yeasts, bacteria, plants, animals, and human beings.

What of the quality of these studies? Ten are unpublished doctoral dissertations, two are masters' theses, and the rest are published primarily in parapsychology journals. These publications have peer

---

*Daniel J. Benor, "Survey of Spiritual Healing Research," *Complementary Medical Research* 4:1, (September 1990): 9–33 and Daniel J. Benor, *Healing Research* (Munich: Helix Verlag GmbH, 1993). Address: Windeckstr. 82, D-81375 Munich, Germany.

review standards as rigorous as many medical journals. These include the *Journal of the American Society for Psychical Research*, the *Journal of Parapsychology*, the *Journal of the Society for Psychical Research*, and the *European Journal of Parapsychology*. *Research in Parapsychology* is a collection of abstracts from the annual meeting of the Parapsychological Association. Its abstracts undergo peer review for conference presentation, although not as rigorous as that of the other journals. The reason researchers in this field do not publish in standard medical journals is that these journals until recently have declined to publish studies in spiritual healing.

Further observations about the quality of research in this field are in Appendix 3.

All references from Benor's survey are provided in the "Reference to Tables 1.1–1.13." Interested readers may pursue the original studies through references 3 through 82, or in Benor's *Healing Research*.

TABLE 1.1 **Controlled trials of healing**

SUBJECT	NO. OF TRIALS	SIGNIFICANT RESULTS*		
Water	5	3		
Crystallization	2	?		
Enzymes	10	3	(+2)	
Fungus/yeast	7	4	(+1)	
Bacteria	10	2		(+3?)
Red blood cells	2	2		
Cancer cells	5	3		(+1?)
Snail pacemaker cells	4	4		
Plants	19	4	(+6)	(+1?)
Motility				
flagellates	3			(+1?)
algae	1			(+1?)
moth larvae	1	1		

*Significance p<.01 or (.02<p<.05) or (?) questionable   *continued on next page*
© Daniel J. Benor, M.D.

Subject	No. of Trials		Significant Results*		
Mice					
skin wounds	2		2		
retard goiter growth	2		2		
malaria	2			(+1)	
tumors decrease	3		1		(+1?)
increase	1		0		
anesthesia	14		10	(+4)	
Chicks malaria	1				(+1?)
Humans					
allobiofeedback	7		2	(+2)	
pre-recorded	1		0		
hemoglobin increase	4		4		
skin wounds	1		1		
hypertension	3		1	(+1)	
asthma/bronchitis	1		0		
coronary care	1		1		
myopia	1				(+1?)
epilepsy	1		?		
leukemia		(1?)	?		
tension headache	1		1		
postoperative pain	1		0		
anxiety	8		4	(+2)	
distant healing sensations	1		1		
personal relationship	1		0		
self-esteem	1			(+1)	
diagnosis	4	(+1?)	0	(+1)	(+1?)
TOTALS	131	(+2?)	56	(+21)	(+11?)

TABLE 1.2 **Healing action on enzymes**

Subject of Healing	Researchers	T/N/D*	Duration	Healer	Results		Significance
Trypsin	J. Smith	T/N	Up to 2 mins	Estebany	Activity increased 10% over 75 mins		Significant (?)
Nicotinamide adenine dinucleotide (NAD)		T/N			Activity decreased		
Amylase - Amylose		T/N			No effect		
			to 3 hrs	Magnet	3,000–13,000 gauss		
Trypsin	Edge	T/N	?	Graham	1. Undamaged trypsin activity increased in one of five studies Combining results of 5 runs		p<.05 p<.01
					2. Trypsin damaged by UV light		NS**
				Magnet	3. Trypsin + magnetic field 1,300 gauss		3/6 runs Significant
Dopamine	Rein	N	15 mins	2 Healers	Increased up to 130% in five mice, decreased down to 25% in five mice		p<.01
Noradrenaline					Increased up to 130% in 5/10 mice		p<.05
Human platelet monoamine oxidase (MAO)	Rein	T/N	4-5 mins	Manning	Increased in 9 trials; decreased in 7; no response in 2		p<.001
Carbondioxydeanhydratase	Kief	N	2 mins	?			NS
Human serum	Frydychowski, et al.	N?	?	2 Healers	Photon emission increased in individual treatments		NS

*T/N/D: Touch/Near/Distant   **NS: Non-Significant

TABLE 1.3 **Healing effects on fungus and yeasts**

Subject of Healing	Researchers	T/N/D*	Duration	Healer	Results	Significance
Fungus	Barry	N	15 mins	10 Healers	5 dishes each—to decrease growth Decreased in 33/39 trials Decreased by 10/11 subjects (some combined efforts) Decreased in 151/194 dishes	p<.001 p<.01 p<.001
Fungus	Tedder & Monty	D	Minimum 5–15 mins/day	7 Healers	3 sess/wk, 3x/sess, 5 cultures/trial Grp. 1. Familiar with researcher—16/16 with 80 dishes, decreased almost 2 mm/dish Grp. 2. Unknown to or infrequent interactions with researchers—4 hits; 11 misses; 3 ties	p<.00006 p<.08
Fungus	Soidla (in Zhukoborsky)	T/N	20 secs 40 secs	Kulagina	Increased nos. of spores: 26 vs. Control: 11 +/– 3 Return to baseline	? ?
			20 secs	Alex. Sh.	18 spores	?
			20 secs	Zhukoborsky	20 spores	?
Yeast	Haraldsson & Thorsteinson	N	?	3 Healers, 4 "Others"	10 test tubes each, 12 sessions Combined results Healers Non-healers	 p<.02 p<.0004 NS**
Yeast	Grad (1965)	T/N vehicle	30 mins	2 Healers	CO_2 production in 16 test tubes; 3/5 sets	p<.0005
Yeast	Cahn & Muscle	T/N	10 mins	Healer	Oxygen production after cyanide poisoning of yeast culture: rate increased with healing	p<.02
Yeast	Nash & Nash	T/N	30 mins	19 psychotics	12 fermentation tubes each to inhibit	Marginal

© Daniel J. Benor, M.D.

*T/N/D: Touch/Near/Distant   **NS: Non-Significant

TABLE 1.4 **Healing effects on bacteria**

Subject of Healing	Researchers	T/N/D*	Duration	Healer	Results	Significance
Bacteria E. Coli	Nash (1982)	D	?	60 subjects	9 test tubes each: 3 to increase vs Controls vs Decrease 3 to decrease vs Controls 3 Controls—left alone	p<.05 p<.001 p<.02
	Li-Da	?	?	Qi Gong Masters	Healing increased growth 700–1,000% Killing decreased growth 50%	? ?
	Leikam	N	?	23 students	Near: Increased 7.5% vs Control Distant: Increased 3.2% vs Control	? ?
Salmonella typhimurium	Rauscher & Rubik	T/N	2 mins	Olga Worrall	1. Phenol inhibition of motility Healed: 93% inhibited in 12 mins Controls: 100% inhibited in 2 mins	? ?
					2. Increased growth phase during active (mid-log, growth) phase NR of growth during inactive (lag) phase	? ?
					3. Protecting bacteria from antibiotics (by dose) Tetracycline 1 mcg: +121% 10 mcg: +28% Chloramphenicol 10 mcg: +70% 100 mcg: +22%	? ? ? ?
					4. Controls hand-warmed by non-healer: +0%	
					5. Tetracycline: more survivors at all times Chloramphenicol: at small generation times, Controls grow better; at large generation times, healed grow better	?

continued on next page

TABLE 1.4 **Healing effects on bacteria** *continued*

Subject of Healing	Researchers	T/N/D*	Duration	Healer	Results	Significance
					6. Sodium nitrate .05 M. (mutagen attacking DNA) decreases viability: −50%	?
					Sodium nitrate + antibiotic increases growth:	
					Tetracycline +50%	?
					Chloramphenicol: +75%	?
Bacterial mutation (growth?) E. Coli	Nash (1984)	D	?	52 ungifted volunteers	Promotion of mutation from lac negative to lac positive; inhibition of same: Controls; (3 test tubes each):	
					Promoted vs inhibited	p<.005
					Inhibited vs controls	p<.02
					Promoted vs controls	NS**

*T/N/D: Touch/Near/Distant   **NS: Non-Significant

TABLE 1.5 **Healing effects on cells in vitro**

SUBJECT OF HEALING	RESEARCHERS	T/N/D*	DURATION	HEALER	RESULTS	SIGNIFICANCE
Red blood cells	Braud, Davis & Wood	9N; 1D	5 mins	Manning	Decreased rate of hemolysis 10 runs, 5 samples each	p<.001
	Braud (1988)	D	1 min	Unselected	32 volunteers each visualized protection to 10 tubes vs 10 Controls	p<.00002
Mouse leukemia	Snel	N	?	Manning	1. Inhibiting growth: Experimental and Controls All cells died	
		D	?		2. +39% Experimental vs Control	p<.002
		N	?	Many people	3. +27.5% Experimental vs Control	.002<p<.02
		D		Manning	4. −18.5% Experimental vs Control	.002<p<.02
Cervical cancer cells	Knetz (From Braud, Davis & Wood)	N & D	20 mins	Manning	Cells adhere to plastic surface of flask electrostatically: 200–1,200% change	?
Snail pacemaker cells	Baumann, Lagle & Roll	N	?	Parapsychologist	1. 1/3 series: increased firing rate, despite intent to decrease it	p<.002
				Healer	2. 1/2 series: decreased rate	p<.01
				Healer	3. 1 series: decreased rate	p<.01
				RSPK agent	4. 4/4 series: decreased rate	.002<p<.01
Chlamydomonas engameba	Alexandrov (Zhukoborsky)	?	5 mins	6 healers	Protection from heat stress, perhaps tolerating 46 degrees vs 43 degrees	?

© Daniel J. Benor, M.D.

*T/N/D: Touch/Near/Distant

TABLE 1.6 **Healing effects on motility of simple organisms**

Subject of Healing	Researchers	T/N/D*	Duration	Healer	Results	Significance
Paramecia	Richmond	N	15 secs	Richmond	1. 794 Experimental (E) vs 799 Control (C): Motility measured in predicted and opposite directions	"Highly Significant"
					2. 701 E vs 701 C	
Stylonychia mytilus	Randall	N	?	Randall	280 E vs 280 C	NS**
Algae	Pleass & Dey	N	4–5 mins	?	Motility, speed influenced	Significant
Lepidoptera (moth) larvae	Metta	?	?	1 subject	4 series: 3 significantly positive; 1 negative Mean Negative series	p<.012 p<.0006
				1 subject		NS

© Daniel J. Benor, M.D.

*T/N/D: Touch/Near/Distant   **NS: Non-Significant

TABLE 1.7 **Healing effects on plants**

Subject of Healing	Researchers	T/N/D*	Duration	Healer	Results	Significance
Barley seeds	Grad (1965)	T/ vehicle	15 mins	Estebany	Barley seeds, damaged by 1% saline solution; decreased damage with healing to the solution	p<.001
					Repeated × 3 with careful blinds, sealed jars of water	.02<p<.05
Rye grass	Macdonald, Hickman, & Dakin	T/ vehicle	20 mins	Kraft	Seeds damaged with healer-treated saline Day 9: total E height less than C 9: mean height less than C 10: mean height less than C	p<.05 p<.02 p<.001
				Worrall	15: total height greater than C 16: total height greater than C 17: mean height greater than C 18: total height greater than C	p<.05 p<.05 p<.05 p<.05
Wheat seeds	Saklani	T	43 secs	Shaman	Treated seeds Mean length greater than C: Days 15–18 14, 19	p<.01 p<.05
		T + T/ vehicle	30 secs	Shaman	Total no. germinating/pot greater than C Mean length greater than C: Days 12 7, 9, 11	p<.01 p<.01 p<.05
Radish seeds	Nicholas	N	15–20 min × 30 days	Nicholas	Weight treated greater than Control Height treated greater than Control	p<.02 NS**
Mung beans	Barrington	T/N	?	Manning	More radicles and plumials vs Control by 7 days	p<.02

continued on next page

*T/N/D: Touch/Near/Distant   **NS: Non-Significant
© Daniel J. Benor, M.D.

TABLE 1.7 **Healing effects on plants** *continued*

Subject of Healing	Researcher	T/N/D*	Duration	Healer	Results	Significance
Rye grass	Miller	T/vehicle	?	?	Sprouting: Controls 8% / Healed 63% / Magnet-Treated 60% Blade growth: 2.8ins / 2.9ins / 3.6ins (avg)	? ?
Corn seeds	Solfvin	D	?	Healer	Checkerboard distribution	NS**
?	Barros, et al	T&D	?	?	Greater growth with distant than touch healing	"more sig."
Corn seeds	Wallack	T/N	30 mins	?	15 seeds at 48, 96 hours root growth	NS
Radish seeds	Lenington	vehicle	?	holy water	12 seeds	NS
Grass seeds	Pauli	D	?	school children	Greater growth when males, females worked apart	?
Barley seeds	Grad (1967)	T/vehicle	7–9 days	depressed	Seeds oven-dried, watered with saline 1 person with neurotic depression vs Control 1 person with psychotic depression vs Control 1 person with "green thumb" vs Control	 sl. more NS significant
Potatoes	Russell	D	?	?	Increase vs untreated Control +32.2%	?
Corn					Increase vs sprayed Control +13.1%	?
					59 treated vs 132 Control infested with borers	?

*T/N/D: Touch/Near/Distant   **NS: Non-Significant

TABLE 1.8 **Effects of healing on animals**

Subject of Healing	Researchers	T/N/D*	Duration	Healer	Results	Significance
Mice Skin wounds	Grad (1965)	N	15 mins ×2/day × 14 days	Estebany	1. 48 mice, more rapid wound healing, day 14	$p<.001$
	Grad, Cadoret & Paul				2. 150 mice, double blinds: days 15, 16	$p<.01$
Retardation of goiter growth	Grad (1965)	1. N	15 mins × 2/day × 5 d/wk × 8 wks	Estebany	1. 23 mice, slower thyroid growth, with baseline and heat controls	$p<.001$
		vehicle	1 hr ×2/ day ×6d/wk		2. 37 mice, same	$p<.001$
Malaria	Solfvin (1982)	D	(?)	3 + (?)	1. 12 mice each 2 believers, 1 non-believer, opposite direction from the expected for: malaria healing	NS** $p<.02$ NS
				5 + (?)	2. 12 mice each: malaria healing	$.05<p<.10$ $p<.05$
Chicks Malaria	Baranger & Filer	Collars	Constant	Metal, vegetable materials	368 chicks wore collars of various metals or plant fibers. Gold, iron, & copper were most effective against malaria	NS
Mice Tumors	Onetto & Elguin	?	?	Elguin	1. 30 Tumorogenic mice, healer to decrease tumor	$.001<p<.01$
					2. Same, healer to increase tumor growth	NS
	Null	T&D	?	50 healers	1. 1 mouse each for E and C 12.8 days (E) vs 8.9 days (C) —44% longer	?
				Weisman	2. 20 mice, 1/2 dose cancer cells 14.9 days (E) vs 12.9 (C) —15.5% longer	?

*T/N/D: Touch/Near/Distant   **NS: Non-Significant

© Daniel J. Benor, M.D

TABLE 1.9 **Healing effects on anaesthetised mice**

RESEARCHERS	T/N/D*	HEALER	RESULTS	SIGNIFICANCE
Watkins & Watkins	D	12 subjects (9 psychic)	1. Experimental mice & healers in one room; Control mice in another: sleep time ***"hits" 157/240	p<.036 p<.01–.001
			2. All in same room: sleep time hits 116/168	p<.001 p<.01
			3. Healers in one room, both mice in another, behind one-way mirror: sleep time hits 237/360	p<.001 p<.001
			Overall results for experiments 1–3	p<.00001
Wells & Klein	D	4 gifted	Per (3) above: 1 experimenter selecting mice, other experimenters testing: sleep time hits 110/192	p<.02–.05 p<.05
Watkins, Watkins & Wells	D	2 gifted psychics	1. One-way mirror, experimenters blind: half-series alternating sides of table, 15–30 minute breaks between halves	p<.026
			2. Mice paired by similar waking times	p<.002
		Non-gifted	3. Believers in ESP vs non-believers Confident vs non-confident	p<.05 p<.01
			4. Healer physiological parameters: GSR Increases in pulse; respiration; skeletal muscle tension; female EKG T wave at end Decreases in pulse amplitude; male EKG T wave at end Waking of paired mice	NS*** } All Significant p<.004
			5. Automatic timing of arousal	p<.00003
			6. Lag effect with random sides for 1/2–runs	p<.002–3
			7. Different experimenters for second 1/2–runs, automatic timing of arousal	p<.04–5

continued on next page

*T/N/D: Touch/Near/Distant   ***"hits": successful trials   ***NS: Non-Significant:

© Daniel I. Benor. M.D.

TABLE 1.9 **Healing effects on anaesthetised mice** *continued*

Researchers	T/N/D*	Healer	Results	Significance
Wells & Watkins	N D(?)		1. Sides randomly chosen, constant in runs: First 1/2 – healers present Second 1/2 – healers left building	p<.002 p<.001
			2. Separate experimenters for each 1/2, second one blind to first-half side: First 1/2 – healers present Second 1/2 – healers left building	p<.024 p<.015–.05
Schlitz	D	3	TV monitors; random number generator for target choice; healer in remote room; arousal time by photo cells: Only 1 healer hit vs miss	p<.05

*T/N/D: Touch/Near/Distant

TABLE 1.10 **Healing effects on electrodermal activity**

SUBJECT OF HEALING	RESEARCHERS	T/N/D*	DURATION	HEALER	RESULTS	SIGNIFICANCE
Humans Allobiofeedback Electrodermal Activity (EDA) or Galvanic Skin Response (GSR)	Braud (1979)	D	30 secs	Manning & 10 others	1. 10 trails each	p<.002
					2. 13 pre-recorded series	NS**
	Braud & Schlitz (1983)	D		Braud & Schlitz	1. 16 people, active GSR vs Controls inactive	p<.015
					2. 16 people, active vs chance	p<.014
					3. 16 people, inactive vs chance	NS

	Braud, et al.
	(1984)
		D		24	1. 24 people, 1/2 feedback; 1/2
					  non-feedback
					  feedback vs non-feedback
						NS

					non-, pre-, and post-intervention	p<.04
					combined pre- vs post- intervention	p<.04
				2 "blind"	2. 16 people cooperating; 16 blocking mentally	NS

				3	3. 5 calm people each; intention
					  to decrease EDA without
					  affecting pulse, temperature,
					  respiration.
					  One healer succeeded on pulse
						p<.02

	Schlitz & Braud	D	20 secs	3	5 sessions, 10 times/session, calm	NS

*T/N/D: Touch/Near/Distant   **NS: Non-Significant

© Daniel J. Benor, M.D.

TABLE 1.11 **Healing effects of human physical problems**

SUBJECT OF HEALING	RESEARCHERS	T/N/D*	DURATION	HEALER	RESULTS	SIGNIFICANCE
Hemoglobin (Hgb) increase	Krieger	T/N	15 mins	Estebany	1. 19 patients, pre- vs post-healing Hgb levels	p<.02
					9 Controls, pre- vs post-time Hgb levels	NS**
					Healed vs Controls Hgb levels	p<.01
					2. 43 healing vs 33 Controls	p<.01
					3. 46 healing vs 33 Controls, matching for diet, breathing exercises, medications	p<.001
		T/N	?	32 nurses	4. 2 patients each, one healing and one Control	
					Healed: pre- vs post-treatment Hgb levels	p<.001
					Controls: pre- vs post-time Hgb levels	NS
Skin wound healing	Wirth	N	5 mins	TT	23 healing vs 21 Controls, days 8 and 16	p<.001
Hypertension	Miller	D	?	8 healers	48 hypertensives, healing added to conventional treatments: Decreased systolic blood pressure	p<.014
	Beutler, et al.	T&D	20 mins	12 healers	All healing & Control patients improved equally Touch healing: greater subjective improvement	p<.005
	Kuang, et al.	Qigong (TT?)	?	?	244 hypertensives, mortality over 0.5–30 years: Qigong 19% (47/244) vs Control 42% (130/312)	p<.01
					Q. consistent 11% vs Q. non-consistent 29%	p<.001
					Hypotensors alone	p<.05
					Controls vs Q. non-consistent	NS

continued on next page

T/N/D: Touch/Near/Distant   **NS: Non-Significant

© Daniel J. Benor, M. D.

TABLE 1.11 **Healing effects of human physical problems** continued

Subject of Healing	Researchers	T/N/D*	Duration	Healer	Results	Significance
Asthma/Asthmatic bronchitis	Attevelt	T&D	15 mins	healers	30 each, T, D, & Controls, pre- vs post-healing. No significant differences between groups	All Sig. Improved
Coronary care	Byrd	D	?	prayer groups	192 healing / 201 Control Antibiotics 3 / 16 Pulmonary edema 6 / 18 Intubation 0 / 12	$p<.005$ $p<.03$ $p<.002$
Myopia	Guo & Ni	T?N?	?	Qigong	30 children 20 Controls: Improved 20 placebo eyedrops NS 20 self-healing NS 2 20 Qigong Master healing 16	?
Epilepsy	Purska-Rowinska & Rejmer	?	?	Healer	42 patients: decreased severity	?
Leukemia	Collipp	D	?	Prayer group	Healing: 10 lymphatic leukemia Control: 6 lymphatic, 2 myelogenous	NS**

*T/N/D: Touch/Near/Distant   **NS: Non-Significant

TABLE 1.12 **Healing effects on subjective sensations**

Subject of Healing	Researchers	T/N/D*	Duration	Healer	Results	Significance
Tension headache	Keller & Bzdek	N	5 mins	TT Healers	30 patients: pain pre- and 4 hrs post-healing	p<.005
					TT vs Mock TT	NS**
					TT vs Mock TT (eliminating 5 TT and 15 MTT who took other treatments during the 4 hrs)	.005<p<.01
Postoperative pain	Meehan	T/N	?	TT Healers	36 each: TT, MTT, & Control (standard treatment)	
					TT vs MTT	NS
					Controls better than TT	Significant
Healee sensations	Goodrich	D		6 LeShan	Synchronous vs non-synchronous healings	p<.005
Personal relationship	Winston	T&D	5 mins	4 LeShan	16 healees rotated through various patterns of familiarity with healers	NS
Anxiety (state)	Heidt	T	5 mins	TT Healer	Cardiac ICU patients:	
					30 pre- vs post-TT	p<.001
					30 TT vs 30 casual touch	p<.01
					30 TT vs 30 no touch	p<.01
	Quinn	N	5 mins	4 TT Healers	Cardiac ICU patients:	
					30 TT vs 30 Mock TT	p<.0005
	Ferguson	T	?	50 & 50 TT Healers	Healees pre- vs post-healing:	
					Experienced healers	p<.0001
					Inexperienced healers	p<.001
					Experienced vs inexperienced healers	p<.001
	Fedoruk	N	25 mins	TT Healers	17 premature infants, pre- vs post-stress + TT	
					Assessment of Premature Infant Behavior	p<.05
					Physiological measure	NS
					Mock TT (suggestive increase)	NS

continued on next page

*T/N/D: Touch/Near/Distant   **NS: Non-Significant

© Daniel J. Benor, M. D.

TABLE 1.12 **Healing effects on subjective sensations** *continued*

Subject of Healing	Researchers	T/N/D*	Duration	Healer	Results	Significance
Anxiety (state)	Collins	T	7 mins	TT Healer	24 TT and Mock TT (all had both treatments) Both groups had decreases in temperature, pulse, and GSR (no between-group significance)	p<.05
	Gulak	?	15 mins	Gulak	76 healees improved	.001<p<.01
	Randolph	T	13 mins	TT Healer	30 college students stressed with movie: GSR, muscle tension, skin temperature	NS**
	Parkes	N	5 mins	TT Healer	20 hospitalized patients, age 65-93, 45 illnesses TT and Mock TT both *increased* anxiety	NS
Self-esteem	Schutze	D	?	Prayer	10 healing vs 27 Control	p<.05

*T/N/D: Touch/Near/Distant   **NS: Non-Significant

TABLE 1.13 **Clairvoyant diagnosis**

RESEARCHERS	DIAGNOSTICIAN		RESULTS	SIGNIFICANCE
Mison	Biodiagnosticians	8	45–85% congruence with physicians' diagnoses (mean 59%)	?
Brier, et al.	Silva Mind Control	5 1	1. 5 diagnoses each 2. One of the 5	NS* p<.05
Vaughan	Silva Mind Control	21	5 patients each diagnosed by the 21 SMC graduates	NS
Shealy	1 each: clairvoyant, graphologist, astrologer, palmist, & psychologist		25–80% accurate, specially the clairvoyant	?
Jacobson & Wicklund	Mind Dynamic	1	10 names, 10 diagnoses	NS

*Non-Significant   © Daniel J. Benor, M. D.

REFERENCES TO TABLES 1.1–1.13

1. Gardner, R. Miracles of healing in Anglo-Celtic Northumbria as recorded by the Venerable Bede and his contemporaries: a reappraisal in the light of twentieth-century experience. *Br. Med. J.* (1983); 287: 1927–33.

2. LeShan L. *The Medium, The Mystic and the Physicist.* New York: Ballantine. (British ed: *Clairvoyant Reality.* Wellingborough, Northants: Thorsons), 1974.

3. Attevelt, J.R.M. *Research into Paranormal Healing.* Ph.D. dissertation, Univ. Utrecht, 1988.

4. Barington, M.R. Bean growth promotion pilot experiment. *Proc. Soc. Psychical Res.* (1982); 56: 302–4.

5. Barros, A., *et al.* Methodology for research on psychokinetic influence over the growth of plants. *Psi Communication* (1977); 3(5/6): 9–30. (Abstract translated from Spanish, in: *Parapsychol. Abstr. Int.* [1984]; 1[2]: 80.)

6. Barry J. General and comparative study of the psychokinetic effect on a fungus culture. *J. Parapsychol.* (1968); 32: 237–43.

7. Baumann. S., Lagle, J., Roll, W. Preliminary results from the use of two novel detectors for psychokinesis. *Res. Parapsychol. 1985* (1986): 59–62.

8. Beutler, J.J., *et al.* Paranormal healing and hypertension. *Br. Med. J.* (1988); 297: 1491–94.

9. Braud, W.G. Allobiofeedback: immediate feedback for a psychokinetic influence upon another person's physiology. *Res. Parapsychol. 1977* (1978): 123–4.

10. Braud, W. Conformance behavior involving living systems. *Res. Parapsychol. 1978*, (1979): 111–5.

11. Braud, W. Distant mental influence of rate of hemolysis of human red blood cells *Res Parapsychol. 1988* (1989): 1–6.

12. Braud, W., Davis, G., Wood, R. Experiments with Matthew Manning. *J. Soc. Psychical. Res.* (1979); 50 (782): 199–223.

13. Braud, W., Schlitz, M. Psychokinetic influence on electrodermal activity. *J. Parapsychol.* (1983); 47(2): 95–119.

14. Braud, W., *et al.* Further studies of the bio-PK effects: feedback, blocking, specificity/generality. *Presentation at Parapsychological Association Meeting,* 1984.

15. Brier, R. PK on a bio-electrical system. *J. Parapsychol.* (1969); 33: 187–205.

16. Brier, R., Savits, B., Schmeidler, G. Tests of Silva Mind Control graduates. *Res. Parapsychol. 1973* (1974): 13–15.

17. Cahn, H., Muscle, N. Toward standardization of "laying-on" of hands investigation. *Psychoenergetic Systems,* (1976); 1: 115–18.

18. Campbell, A. "Treatment" of tumors by PK. *J Soc. Psychical Res.* (1968); 46: 428.

19. Collins, J.W. *The Effect of Non-Contact Therapeutic Touch on the Relaxation Response.* Unpublished master's thesis, Vanderbilt Univ., Nashville, Tennessee, 1983.

20. Collip, P.J. The efficacy of prayer: a triple-blind study. *Med. Tim.* (1969); 97(5): 201–4.

21. Di Liscia, J.C. Psychic healing: an attempted investigation. *Psi Communicacion* (1977); 3(5/6): 101–10. (Abstract translated from Spanish, in *Parapsychol. Abstr. Int.* [1984]; 2(1): 82.)

22. Edge. H. The effect of laying on of hands on an enzyme: an attempted replication. *Res. Parapsychol. 1979* (1980); 137–39.

23. Fedoruk, R.B. *Transfer of the Relaxation Response: Therapeutic Touch as a Method for the Reduction of Stress in Premature Neonates.* Unpublished Ph.D. dissert., Univ. Maryland, 1984.

24. Ferguson, C.K. *Subjective Experience of Therapeutic Touch (SETTS): Psychometric Examination of an Instrument.* Unpublished Ph.D. dissert., Univ. Maryland, 1984.

25. Frydrychowski, A.F., Przyjemska, B., Orlowski, T. An attempt to apply photon emission measurement in the selection of the most effective healer. (Translated from Polish by A. Imich) *Psychotronika* (1985): 82–83.

26. Goodrich, J. *Psychic Healing—a Pilot Study.* Unpublished Ph.D. dissert., Union Graduate School, Yellow Springs, Ohio, 1974.

27. Grad, B. A telekinetic effect on plant growth: I. *Int. J. Parapsychol.* (1963); 5: 117–34.

28. Grad, B. A telekinetic effect on plant growth: II. Experiments involving treatment of saline in stoppered bottles. *Int. J. Parapsychol.* (1964); 6: 473–98.

29. Grad, B. A telekinetic effect on plant growth: III. Stimulating and inhibiting effects. Res. brief presented to the *Seventh Annual Convention of the Parapsychological Association,* Oxford Univ., 1964.

30. Grad, B. Some biological effects of laying-on of hands: a review of experiments with animals and plants. *J Amer. Soc. Psychical Res.* (1965); 59: 95–127.

31. Grad, B. PK effects of fermentation of yeast. *Proc. Parapsychol. Assoc.* (1965); 2: 15–16.

32. Grad, B. The "laying on of hands" implications for psychotherapy, gentling, and the placebo effect. *J. Soc. Psychical Res.* (1967); 61(4): 286–305.

33. Grad, B., Cadoret, R.J., Paul, G.I. The influence of an unorthodox method of treatment on wound healing in mice. *Int. J. Parapsychol.* (1961); 3: 5–24.

34. Guo and Ni. Studies of Qi Gong in treatment of myopia. In *Encounters with Qi,* edited by D. Eisenberg. New York: Norton, 1985; pp. 202–3.

35. Heidt, P. *An Investigation of the Effect of Therapeutic Touch on the Anxiety of Hospitalized Patients.* Unpublished Ph.D. dissert., New York Univ., 1979.

36. Joyce, C.R.B., Welldon, T.M.C. The objective efficacy of prayer: a double-blind clinical trial. *J. Chron. Dis.* (1965); 18: 367–77.

37. Keller, E., Bzkek, V.M. Effects of Therapeutic Touch on tension headache pain. *Nurs. Res.* (1986): 101–4.

38. Kief, H.K. A method for measuring PK with enzymes. *Res. Parapsychol. 1972* (1973): 19–20.

39. Krieger, D. Therapeutic Touch: the imprimatur of nursing. *Am. J. Nurs.* (1975); 7: 784–87.

40. Kuang, A.K., *et al.* Long-term observation on Qi gong in prevention of stroke—follow-up of 244 hypertensive patients for 18–22 years. *J. Trad. Chinese Med.* (1986); 6(4): 235–38.

41. Lenington, S. Effects of holy water on the growth of radish plants. *Psychol. Rep.* (1979); 45: 381–82.

42. Li-Da, F. The effects of external Qi on bacterial growth patterns. *China Qi Gong Magazine* (1983); 1: 36. (Cited in: Eisenberg, D. *Encounters with Qi.* New York: Norton, 1985; p. 213).

43. Lionberger, H.J. *An Interpretive Study of Nurses' Practice of Therapeutic Touch*. Unpublished Ph.D. dissert., Univ. California, San Francisco, 1985.

44. Macdonald, R.G., Hickman, J.K., Dakin, H.S. *Preliminary Physical Measurements of Psychophysical Effects Associated with Three Alleged Psychic Healers*. San Francisco: Washington Research Centre research brief, 1976 (July 1).

45. Cardiologist studies effect of prayer on patients. *Med. Trib.* 1986; (Jan 8) (Also in *Brain/Mind Bull.* (1986); 11[7]: 1). These are reports of the original research published later as Byrd, R.C. Positive therapeutic effects of intercessory prayer in a coronary care population. *Southern Med. J.* (1988); 81(7): 826–29.

46. Meehan, T.C. *An Abstract of the Effect of Therapeutic Touch on the Experience of Acute Pain in Post-Operative Patients*. Unpublished Ph.D. dissert., New York Univ., 1985.

47. Metta, L. Psychokinesis on lepidopterous larvae. *J. Parapsychol.* (1972); 36: 213–21.

48. Miller, R.N. Study of remote mental healing. *Med. Hypoth.* (1982); 8: 481–90.

49. Nash, C.B. Psychokinetic control of bacterial growth. *J. Soc. Psychical Res.* (1982); 51: 217–21.

50. Nash CB. Test of psychokinetic control of bacterial mutation. *J. Amer. Soc. Psychical Res.* (1984); 78(2): 145–52.

51. Nash, C.B., Nash, C.S. The effect of paranormally conditioned solution on yeast fermentation. *J. Parapsychol.* (1967); 31: 314.

52. Nicholas, C. The effects of loving attention on plant growth. *New Eng. J. Parapsychol.* (1977); 1: 19–24.

53. Null, G. Healers or hustlers: IV. *Self Help Update* (1981) (Spring); 18.

54. Onetto, B., Elguin, G.H. Psychokinesis in experimental tumorogenesis (Abstract). *J. Parapsychol.* (1966); 30: 220.

55. Parkes, B.S. *Therapeutic Touch as an Intervention to Reduce Anxiety in Elderly Hospitalized Patients*. Unpublished Ph.D. dissert., Univ. Texas at Austin, 1985.

56. Pauli, E. PK on living targets as related to sex, distance, and time. *Res. Parapsychol. 1972* (1973): 68–70.

57. Pleass, C.M., Dey, N.D. Using the Doppler effect to study behavioral responses of motile algae to psi stimulus. *Parapsychol. Assoc. Presented Papers* (1985): 373–405.

58. Quinn, J. *An Investigation of the Effect of Therapeutic Touch without Physical Contact on State Anxiety of Hospitalized Cardiovascular Patients*. Unpublished Ph.D. thesis, New York Univ., 1982.

59. Randall, J.L. An attempt to detect psi effects with protozoa. *J. Soc. Psychical Res.* (1970); 45: 294–96.

60. Randolph, G.L. *The Differences in Psychological Response of Female College Students Exposed to Stressful Stimulus, When Simultaneously Treated by Either Therapeutic Touch or Casual Touch*. Unpublished Ph.D. dissert., New York Univ., 1979.

61. Rauscher, E.A., Rubik, B.A. Effects on motility behavior and growth of salmonella typhimurium in the presence of a psychic subject. *Res. Parapsychol. 1979* (1980): 140–42.

62. Rauscher, E.A., Rubik, B.A. Human volitional effects on a model bacterial system. *Psi Res.* (1983); 2(1): 38–48.

63. Rein, G. *An Exosomatic Effect on Neurotransmitter Metabolism in Mice: a Pilot Study.* Cambridge: 2nd Int. Society for Psychical Research Conference, 1978.

64. Rein, G. A psychokinetic effect of neurotransmitter metabolism: alterations in the degradative enzyme monoamine oxidase. *Res. Parapsychol. 1985* (1986): 77–80.

65. Richmond, N. Two series of PK tests on paramecia. *J. Soc. Psychical Res.* (1952); 36: 577–78.

66. Saklani, A. Preliminary tests for psi-ability in shamans of Garkwal Preliminary. *J. Soc. Psychical Res.* (1988); 55(81): 60–70.

67. Schlitz, M. *PK on Living Systems: Further Studies with Anaesthetized Mice.* SE Regional Parapsychol. Association Presentation, 1982. (Reviewed in Weiner, D.H. Report of 1982 SERPA Conference. *Parapsychol. Rev.* (1982); 13[4]: 13.)

68. Schlitz, M.J., Braud, W.G. Reiki plus natural healing: an ethnographic/experimental study. *Psi Res.* (1985); 4(3/4): 100–23. (Also in *Res. Parapsychol. 1985* [1986]: 17–18.)

69. Smith, J. Paranormal effects on enzyme activity. *Human Dimensions* (1972); 1: 15–19.

70. Snel, F.W.J. PK influence on malignant cell growth. *Res. Letter, Univ. Utrecht* (1980); 10: 19–27.

71. Solfvin, G.F. Studies of the effects of mental healing and expectations on the growth of corn seedlings. *Eur. J. Parapsychol.* (1982); 4(3): 287–323.

72. Solfvin, G.F. Psi expectancy effects in psychic healing studies with malarial mice. *Eur. J. Parapsychol.* (1982); 4(2): 160–97.

73. Tedder, W., Monty, M. Exploration of long-distance PK: a conceptual replication of the influence on a biological system. *Res. Parapsychol. 1980* (1981); 90–93.

74. Vaughan, A. Investigation of Silva Mind Control claims. *Res. Parapsychol. 1973* (1974); 51.

75. Wallack, J.M. Testing for the psychokinetic effect on plants: effect of a "laying on" of hands on germinating corn seed. *Psychological Rep.* (1984); 55: 15–18.

76. Watkins, G.K., Watkins, A.M. Possible PK influence on the resuscitation of anesthetized mice. *J. Parapsychol.* (1971); 35(4): 257–72.

77. Watkins, G.K., Watkins, A.M., Wells, R.A. Further studies on the resuscitation of anaesthetized mice. *Res. Parapsychol. 1972* (1973): 157–59.

78. Wells, R., Klein, J. A replication of a "psychic healing" paradigm. *J. Parapsychol.* (1972); 36: 144–47.

79. Wells, R., Watkins, G. Linger effects in several PK experiments. *Res. Parapsychol. 1974* (1975): 143–47.

80. Winston, S. *Research in Psychic Healing: a Multivariate Experiment.* Unpublished Ph.D. dissert., Union Graduate School, Yellow Springs, Ohio, 1975.

81. Wirth, D. *The Effect of Noncontact Therapeutic Touch on the Healing Rate of Full Thickness Dermal Wounds.* Master's thesis, JFK University, California, 1989.

82. Zhukoborsky, S. An experimental approach to the study of psychic healing. In *Parapsychology in the USSR, Part III,* edited by L. Villenskaya. San Francisco: Washington Research Center, 1981; pp. 52–54.

83. Edge, H.L., *et al. Foundations of Parapsychology.* Boston & London: Routledge & Kegan Paul, 1986.

84. Nash, C.B. *Parapsychology.* Springfield, Ill: Thomas, 1986.

85. Benor, D.J. Lamarckian genetics: evidence from psi research and the work of Luther Burbank. *Res. Parapsychol. 1987* (1988): 166–70.

86. Loehr, F. *The Power of Prayer on Plants.* New York: Signet, 1969.

87. Krieger, D. *The Therapeutic Touch.* Englewood Cliffs, NJ: Prentice Hall, 1979.

88. Chesi, G. *Voodoo.* Worgl, Austria: Perlinger, 1980.

89. Long, M.F. *Recovering the Ancient Magic.* Cape Girardeau, MO: Huna, 1978.

90. Slomoff, D.A. *Voodoo Healing.* Proc. 2nd International Conference Study on the Study of Shamanism. Berkeley: Univ. California, Center S and SE Asia Studies, 1985.

91. Mison, K. *Statistical Processing of Diagnostics Done by Subject and by Physician.* Proc, 6th International Conference Psychotronic Research, 1986; pp. 137–38.

92. Shealy, C.N. The role of psychics in medical diagnosis. In *Frontiers of Science and Medicine,* edited by R. Carlson. London: Wildwood House; pp. 129–37.

93. Kiskos, J. Personal Communication, 1989.

94. Dean, D. *An Examination of Infra-red and Ultra-violet Techniques for Changes in Water Following the Laying-on of Hands.* Unpublished Ph.D. dissert., Saybrook Institute, CA, 1983.

95. Dean, D., Brame, E. *Physical Changes in Water by Laying-on of Hands.* Proc. 2nd International Conference Psychotronic Research, 1975; pp. 200–201.

96. Miller, R. Methods of detecting and measuring healing energies. In *Future Science,* edited by J. White and S. Krippner. Garden City, NY: Anchor/Doubleday, 1977.

97. Miller, R.N. *The Relationship Between the Energy State of Water and Its Physical Properties.* Los Angeles: Ernest Holmes Research Foundation Report (undated).

98. Patrovsky, V. On the bioactivation of water. *Int. J. Paraphysics* (1978); 12(5/6): 130–32.

99. Schwartz, S.A. *et al. Infrared Spectra Alteration in Water Proximate to the Palms of Therapeutic Practitioners.* Los Angeles: Mobius Society Report, 1986.

Spontaneous Regression of Cancer

This section examines more fully the cases of spontaneous regression of cancer reported in 1975 by Yujiro Ikemi and his colleagues at Kyushu University's School of Medicine in Fukuoka, Japan.[1] These cases are noteworthy because of the apparent role of spirituality in the healing.

THE CASES

Case 1

This case is discussed in chapter 1.

Case 2

K. N. was born on a Japanese farm in 1894. He became a member of a religious organization at age nineteen and was appointed a teacher of a church at age twenty-three. His dedication was exemplary and he was presented a national award for his service.

K. N. developed a feeling of fullness and dull pain in the stomach in April 1970, at the age of seventy-seven. Evaluation, which involved gastroscopy and biopsy of a suspicious area in the stomach, confirmed a diagnosis of adenocarcinoma.

K. N. was advised to undergo gastrectomy (surgical removal of the stomach) but declined. At the time of diagnosis, he was very frustrated. His son, whom he had expected to take over his church duties, had been appointed to lead a church far away. K. N. was disappointed that now he had lost his successor and would have to assume all the demanding church work by himself.

On learning of his diagnosis, he summoned a family council. He informed everyone that he wished to serve God for the remainder of his days, and that he would be satisfied if God took his life at any time. He revealed his wish not to have surgery. He expressed his desire to continue his daily work as well as his custom of drinking sake. All his relatives agreed and approved of him. From that time onward, he complained of fewer stomach symptoms and continued his church work as usual, even traveling for mission work and pilgrimages.

Follow-up gastroscopy and biopsy in 1974 showed that the tumor had spontaneously regressed. At the time of his report in 1975, Ikemi verified that K. N.'s vitality and health were excellent and that he looked ten years younger than he is.

Case 3

K. A., a Japanese housewife, was born on a farm in 1935. She became a member of a religious organization while in high school. At age twenty-four, she married and had a son. Her husband proved to be difficult. He would "go out on his business till late at night," often engaging in extended drinking parties. K. A.'s response was to repress her anger about these problems.

In March 1966 she consulted a physician because of stomach pains, weight loss, and general malaise, which she attributed to an ulcer. An extensive evaluation led to surgery. When the surgeon opened the abdomen he found numerous thumb-sized metastases on the wall of the stomach and lymph nodes. The diagnosis was proved microscopically to be adenocarcinoma. The surgeon removed two-thirds of the stomach and performed a procedure he hoped would prevent obstruction. He closed the abdomen, leaving the metastases otherwise untouched. The cancer was so advanced he informed the family K. A. would live three months at most.

"Frankly speaking," she said, "I was not afraid of cancer. That was because I had my religious faith. But without it, I would have given in to the fear of cancer." She continued,

I suffered from cancer much earlier before reaching what is called "the cancer age." Because of this, I was forced to an early mental awakening. I had been a stubborn person and I feel I had my corners rounded off by having cancer. Faith to me is not the attachment to life just wishing to be saved, but it is the gratitude to god [sic] who saved my spirit. I [began] to live a real life since that time.

Nine years following surgery, she remained in excellent health. Physical examination and X rays showed no remaining evidence of cancer and no signs of metastases.

Case 4

K. K. was born on a farm in 1896 in Japan. At age sixteen he became a believer in the Nichiren sect of Buddhism. He worked as a grade-school teacher for a while, and married at age twenty-eight.

K. K. and his wife lived in Northern China during World War II. On returning to Japan, they found it hard to survive. He raised rice on a farm and she peddled dry goods around the country to make ends meet. Life was extremely difficult and he had no one to turn to for help.

During this state of affairs, while forty-seven years old, he noticed rectal bleeding, which he attributed to hemorrhoids. On examination at the university medical school, however, a ring-shaped cancerous growth was discovered just inside the rectum. The physician recommended surgery but K. K. declined because he could not afford it. This was just following World War II, and Japan's Comprehensive Social Insurance System had not then been established, which meant that he would have had to pay for his surgery from his own pocket. Because he had no one from whom to borrow the huge sum, he decided that he would simply "work hard as long as he could live even if it meant a year or two."

He developed increasing abdominal and back pain and emaciation. Gradually, however, these symptoms began to disappear.

Three decades later—in 1973, at age seventy-six—new symptoms began, including a feeling of stomach fullness. His evaluation, which included a stomach biopsy through the gastrocamera, revealed a highly malignant cancer. Again he refused treatment of all types. At the time of Ikemi's report in 1975, he remained alive and quite well.

K. K. stated that his Buddhist faith was a major strength supporting him during his difficult lifetime. He seemed to embody the Buddhist belief that "attachments" of all sorts are the root of all suffering, for all his life he was distinctly unconcerned about worldly ambitions and achievements.

Case 5

Y. Y. was born in 1920 in Japan and married a farmer at the age of twenty-one. The family into which she married had accumulated a large debt the previous generation, which she was expected to help pay in the hope of regaining the family farm, which had been sold. It was not unusual for her to rise at 4:00 A.M. to work in the fields, going to bed at 1:00 A.M. When she was not working on the farm, she was selling vegetables in the daytime and doing house chores at night. In addition to having a very strict mother-in-law, whom she was expected to obey to the letter, she was married to a dictatorial, self-centered husband. Her ability to repress her negative feelings and simply put up with things rivaled her capacity for hard physical work. Y. Y. later described her life as "bitter as death."

During her unimaginable hardships of more than thirty years, she maintained good health, not even catching cold. However, at age fifty-eight she began to experience abdominal pain, which she ascribed to too much hard work on the farm. She began to lose blood from her intestinal tract and became so weak and anemic she required repeated blood transfusions. Following medical evaluation she underwent abdominal surgery, at which time extensive metastases were found in the region of the stomach and elsewhere in the abdominal cavity. A biopsy found adenocarcinoma of the stomach, and doctors performed a palliative resection of the stomach. Her case was considered hopeless; her family was told she would live only one to three months.

Y. Y. responded to these developments with neither anxiety nor depression. Following surgery she began to regain her strength, and four months later she was discharged from the hospital with steadily improving health.

At the time she became ill, a drastic change in her life began to take place. The attitude of the entire family shifted. She had sacrificed her life to them and they now set her free from these responsibilities. Moreover they began actually to protect her with kindness, love, and sympathetic concern. She also experienced changes in her own attitudes. She gained insight into her "naive, religious-minded personality" and began to question the self-centeredness that previously had dominated her interpersonal relationships. She began to engage in outgoing recreational activities such as taking short trips with her friends. She joined a group involved in reciting Chinese poems, which was an effective outlet for her repressed emotions. Five years following her operation, her health remained excellent and she claimed she still was able to work as hard as any woman.

KEY FEATURES OF THE JAPANESE CANCER CASES

Ikemi and his colleagues were deeply impressed by several common features of these cases.

1. All five patients experienced cancer while suffering from a severe existential crisis. Accepting the responsibility for resolving the crisis for themselves preceded the spontaneous regression of their cancer.

2. They had a remarkable absence of anxiety and depression following their diagnoses. In the first four cases, the patients' passionate religious faith seemed vital in countering these emotional reactions. In the fifth, her previous life was so horrid ("bitter as death") that cancer may have seemed trivial by comparison.

3. All the patients gave themselves totally to the will of God after learning they had cancer. This was not passivity, resignation, or giving up, but rather a commitment leading to a renewed devotion to previous activities or to new interests in life. They seemed to sense a larger plan and a fuller meaning to life's events—including cancer—as if more, not less, was now called from them.

4. All five patients took measures to reconstruct their relationships with others. This meant acknowledging personality traits in themselves that had contributed to their difficulties with others, such as rigidity and self-centeredness.

5. A religious or spiritual point of view was prominent in the lives of these patients, particularly in the first four.

Spontaneous Remission: The Latest Findings

As this book goes to press, the Institute of Noetic Sciences (IONS), of Sausalito, California, has just published the most comprehensive investigation of spontaneous remission ever done—*Spontaneous Remission: An Annotated Bibliography*. This fifteen-year project was the work of biochemist Caryle Hirshberg and researcher Brendan O'Regan, who combed 3,500 references from more than eight hundred journals in twenty languages. This report deals not only with cancer but also with the spontaneous remission of a wide spectrum of diseases. It is the largest database of medically reported cases of spontaneous remission in the world. Key findings:

• Remission is a widely-documented phenomenon, almost certainly commoner than generally believed.

• Remission is an extremely promising area of research. Studying the psychobiological processes involved may provide important clues in understanding the body's self-regulatory processes and the breakdowns that precede the onset of many diseases.

• Data on remissions can have an important influence on how patients are treated and handled when diagnosed with a terminal illness. Restoring "ethical hope" may help instill a "fighting spirit," an important factor in recovery from illness.

Spontaneous Remission: An Annotated Bibliography can be obtained from the Institute of Noetic Sciences, Box 909, Sausalito, California 94966–0909.

How Good Is the Evidence? Prayer, Meditation, and Parapsychology

PRAYER

Prayer has much in common with parapsychology, the field of psychology that examines psychic phenomena such as telepathy and clairvoyance. Prayer also resembles meditation, and cannot be sharply separated from it. Both parapsychology and meditation have been severely criticized by skeptics in recent years, and prayer can expect the same treatment as evidence for its effectiveness becomes more widely known.

Some of the sternest rejections of the type of phenomena examined in this book have come from the National Research Council (NRC), a governmental body often charged with evaluating certain areas within science. In 1988 and 1991 the NRC issued reports dealing with, among other things, meditation and parapsychology[1] Because the conclusions of the NRC reports differ from those of this book, and because these reports have been quite influential in shaping public opinion, I believe it is important to comment on these discrepancies. I hope this will be of value to people interested in prayer when they encounter similar criticisms.

MEDITATION

The 1991 NRC report stated, "Overall, our assessment of the scientific research on meditation (primarily, transcendental meditation [TM]) leads to the conclusion that it seems to be no more effective . . . than are established relaxation techniques; it is unwarranted to attribute any special effects to meditation alone."[2] The NRC report reached this conclusion by drawing primarily on two previous narrative reviews. One of these, by D. S. Holmes, covered less than half the relevant studies in Transcendental Meditation available at the time it was prepared.[3] The other, by J. Brener and S. R. Connally, also appears to have ignored much of the available and relevant research.[4]

Meta-analysis, a powerful analytical tool used by statisticians, allows them essentially to combine many short experiments into one long one. Using this technique they can bring together for statistical analysis studies that address the same question, even though the individual studies may have involved different experimental techniques, had different numbers of subjects, and produced different results. This makes possible an overall quantitative assessment of the strength of the effect being examined.[5] A meta-analysis by TM researchers M.C. Dillbeck and D. W. Orme-Johnson on the effects of meditation came to a different conclusion but was ignored in the NRC report. Their quantitative approach showed that the effect size for TM on basal skin resistance, respiration rate, and plasma lactate was over twice that of resting quietly.[6]

K. R. Eppley, A. I. Abrams, and J. Shear, addressing psychological and physiological measures of anxiety, showed that TM typically produces two or three times the reductions in effects of chronic stress compared with other meditation and relaxation techniques.[7] Yet the NRC report said "no evidence supports the notion that . . . meditation permits a person to better cope with a stressor."

Meta-analysis also allows one to compare the results of studies done by experimenters who are cordial, neutral, and negative toward TM. The Eppley, et al. meta-analysis demonstrated that the positive conclusions reached in studies of TM are not the result of selective reporting, and that the NRC's characterization of researchers who are practitioners of meditation as subjectively biased "devotees" is without merit. The Eppley, et al. meta-analysis also contradicted the Brener and Connally claim that meditation research suffered from "weak design" by providing quantitative demonstration that the results cannot be accounted for by subject selection, experimenter bias, expectancies, or atmospheric effects.

The NRC report embodies some faulty assumptions about meditation. It expresses the expectation that meditation should "[lower] reactivity to challenge," that is, make one less responsive to stressors, perhaps through "distracting a person" or providing a "quiet place." But this is neither the traditional nor the express purpose of TM, which is to achieve "restful alertness, a state of unifying capacity."[8] These misunderstandings may be due to the fact, acknowledged by the NRC, that no one on their committee was personally familiar with the *experience* of any of the meditation practices they reviewed. The committee also acknowledged the difficulties this created: "It seems appropriate to be mindful of the constraints that science, as well as culture, background, and personal life experience, places on how the committee views the field of meditation."[9]

The most glaring omission in the NRC report is a large database (more than forty published reports) of societal impact studies of what the TM researchers call the consciousness field. The theory underlying this research is that the field, when supported by a sufficient number of meditators, produces the effects and benefits of meditation in the larger population. This is a nonlocal effect, a type of action-at-a-distance, and the TM researchers describe a correspondence to aspects of quantum nonlocality in their efforts to explain the results of these studies.

On the positive side, the NRC report makes a number of very sensible recommendations for research. In a general observation they state that "learning to relax and enjoy good feelings may prompt a person to make positive changes in his or her work and personal situation ... it may be that meditation and relaxation ... effect cognitive change."[10]

PARAPSYCHOLOGY

In its 1988 report, the NRC is strongly critical of parapsychology, which deals with nonlocal events such as those exemplified in prayer and spiritual healing. The NRC emphasized their belief that over 130 years of research have failed to find any evidence of parapsychological phenomena.

D. L. Radin and R. D. Nelson reported the largest meta-analysis
of parapsychological findings ever done—a total of 832 studies from
sixty-eight investigators, involving the influence of human consciousness on microelectronic systems.[11] The results: "Radin and Nelson's
meta-analysis demonstrates that the. . . results are *robust* and *repeatable*.
Unless critics want to allege wholesale collusion among more than sixty
experimenters or suggest a methodological artifact common to . . . hundred[s of] experiments conducted over nearly three decades, there is no
escaping the conclusion that [these] effects are indeed possible."[12]

Meta-analysis has also been applied to research studies in precognition, which typically involve card-guessing by a subject *before* the targets are even prepared. C. Honorton and D. C. Ferrari found 309
studies in English-language publications by sixty-two investigators, involving over 50,000 subjects who participated in nearly 2 million trials.
Their findings:

• Thirty percent of the studies produced statistically significant
results (where 5 percent was expected by chance). The odds of this result happening by chance are approximately 1 in 1,024.

• The results could not be explained by failure of researchers to
report negative studies (the "file drawer" effect).

• Studies with the most rigorous methodology tended to produce
better results (exactly the opposite of critics' claims).

• The effect size remained constant over the more than fifty years
under consideration.[13]

One charge frequently made about parapsychology and the nonlocal phenomena we've examined in this book is that the quality of research in these areas is low or substandard. In its 1988 report dealing
with parapsychology, the NRC commissioned psychologist Robert
Rosenthal of Harvard University to prepare an evaluation of several controversial areas, including parapsychology. Parapsychology researcher
Richard S. Broughton describes these events:

Rosenthal is widely regarded as one of the world's experts in evaluating controversial research claims in the social sciences and has
spent much of his career developing techniques to provide objective assessments of conflicting data. Neither Rosenthal nor his

coauthor, Monica Harris, had taken any public position on para-psychology. . . . The report by Harris and Rosenthal determined that the "research quality" of the parapsychology research was the best of all the areas under scrutiny. . . . Incredibly . . . [the] com-mittee chairman . . . asked Rosenthal to withdraw the parapsy-chology section of his report. Rosenthal refused. In the final document the Harris and Rosenthal report is cited only in the several sections dealing with nonparapsychological topics; there is no mention of it in the parapsychology section.[14]

Science is a rough-and-tumble activity that includes robust, healthy debate. But the debate should not only be rigorous, it should be unbiased as well.

Healing and the Mind: A Summing Up

Mind and body can interact in a great variety of ways to bring about health or illness, as we have seen throughout this book. If we take the widest possible view of these interactions, certain patterns emerge, shown in Table 4.1.

TABLE 4.1 **Healing and the Mind**

LOCAL EFFECTS (sensory mediated)				NONLOCAL EFFECTS (nonsensory mediated)	
INTRAPERSONAL		INTERPERSONAL		TRANSPERSONAL	
POSITIVE	NEGATIVE	POSITIVE	NEGATIVE	POSITIVE	NEGATIVE
Conscious and unconscious thoughts, attitudes, emotions, feelings, beliefs, perceived meanings, self-suggestions, images, and visualizations taking place *within* an individual.		Conscious and unconscious suggestions, statements, behaviors, both verbal and nonverbal, taking place *between* individuals.		*Anecdotal evidence:* Distant/psychic/ spiritual healing Intercessory prayer Telesomatic events *Laboratory evidence:* Transpersonal imagery Controlled experiments in humans as well as many nonhuman species involving actual prayer or a prayer-like state ("prayerfulness")	*Anthropological evidence:* Observations of "distant hexing" such as the Polnesian/ Hawaiian "death prayer" *Laboratory evidence:* Many nonhuman species harmed or retarded in controlled experiments

© Larry Dossey, M.D.

As indicated, all known mind-body events are either *local* or *nonlocal* in nature. Local events are mediated by the senses—speech, hearing, touch, smell, sight, and so on—and are describable by the known laws of physics and human physiology. They occur in the here-and-now. They may be *intrapersonal*, occurring within an individual, or *interpersonal*, occurring between two or more people. It is well known that intrapersonal effects may be either positive or negative: our thoughts, attitudes, emotions, and beliefs are a two-edged sword that can heal or harm us. The words and behaviors of others may also either help or harm; thus interpersonal effects may be either positive or negative as well.

The best-known "local, interpersonal, negative" mind-body event is perhaps voodoo. But less dramatic examples are commonplace in medical practice, such as the deplorable habit of physicians called "hanging crepe." The name of this custom is derived from the practice of hanging *black* crepe at morbid events such as funerals. When a doctor "hangs crepe," he paints the very worst picture to the patient. If things turn out the way he predicts, he is wise and is a prophet; if things turn out better, he is a hero and the patient is grateful. In either case, the doctor wins. The ethics of this pernicious custom are questionable. Like voodoo victims, patients can live out dire predictions, sometimes to the extent of dying.

The other major division of mind-body effects is *nonlocal* in nature. Nonlocal mind-body events are initiated between individuals who are too far apart to communicate by the senses. For this reason they are *transpersonal* in nature. They, too, can be either positive or negative. As we have seen, abundant anecdotal evidence supports the existence of "nonlocal, transpersonal, positive" events—distant, psychic, or spiritual healing; the benevolent action of intercessory prayer; and telesomatic events. Laboratory evidence for these happenings also abounds, such as the careful studies in transpersonal imagery and the controlled experiments in humans and nonhumans, examined in part 3 and Appendix 1. And as we saw in chapter 9, a corresponding "dark" side to these events exists—"nonlocal, transpersonal, negative" effects—evidenced by anthropological accounts such as the Polynesian and Hawaiian "death prayer"; and controlled laboratory studies in which living organisms have been harmed, or whose metabolic functions have been retarded.

On close examination we can see that these divisions are not pure states. Consider, for example, the death prayer. It is most commonly initiated by a shaman who is at a great distance from the victim—a decidedly nonlocal, transpersonal event that cannot in principle be explained by sensory mediation. However, when the ascending paralysis and numbness begin, the victim begins to experience fears and other negative thoughts, both consciously and unconsciously, which are local, intrapersonal, and negative in nature. Therefore mind-body events that are initiated nonlocally almost always have local repercussions. This is true for all the examples of nonlocal events we've examined including transpersonal imagery, intercessory prayer, and distant healing.

THE LOCAL EFFECTS OF PRAYER

When you hear hoofbeats in Texas,
think of horses, not zebras.

—Medical school aphorism

Throughout this book we have emphasized the *nonlocal* effects of prayer, such as when an individual prays that a distant person be healed. But it is not necessary to postulate nonlocal mechanisms for many of the healthful effects of prayer.

Jeffrey S. Levin, Ph.D., an epidemiologist at Eastern Virginia Medical School, is the primary architect of an evolving field called the "epidemiology of religion" and is perhaps the most knowledgeable investigator of the *local* effects of prayer and religious practices. But Levin does not discount nonlocal explanations. "I have no doubt that these [nonlocal] mechanisms are real," he states. "I have experienced. . . these types of healing. . . . [But] naturalistic explanations exist [for prayer's healthful effects] which do not require. . . a leap of faith."[1]

In his research, which is supported by a grant from the National Institutes of Health (NIH), Levin has uncovered *over 250 empirical studies* published in the epidemiologic and medical literature since the nineteenth century in which spiritual or religious practices have been statistically associated with particular health outcomes. This literature, "lying forgotten at the margins of medical research," is virtually unknown by physicians and not taught in medical schools. Positive effects for both morbidity and mortality have been found for cardiovascular disease, hypertension, stroke, nearly every type of cancer, colitis, and enteritis. These findings hold regardless of how spirituality is defined and measured, whether according to beliefs, behaviors, attitudes, experiences, and so forth. Over two dozen studies demonstrate the health-promoting effects of simply attending church or synagogue on a regular basis.[2] These benefits have been found to be widely distributed, appearing in studies of Whites, Blacks, and Hispanics; in older adults and adolescents; in U.S., European, African, and Asian subjects; in prospective, retrospective, and case-control studies; in Protestants, Catholics, Jews, Parsis, Buddhists, and Zulus; in studies measuring spirituality as belief in God and religious attendance, among other things; and in studies of self-limiting acute conditions, of fatal chronic diseases, and of illnesses with lengthy, brief, or absent latency periods between exposure and diagnosis and mortality. "In short," Levin states, "something worthy of serious investigation seems to be consistently manifesting in these studies, and understanding the *what*, *how*, and *why* of this apparent spiritual factor in health. . . may be critical for reducing suffering and curing the sick."

How do prayer and spiritual practices act *locally* to influence physical health? There are many possibilities:

• Many spiritual paths or belief systems require certain austerities of the devout which are healthful. Mormons, Seventh-day Adventists, and Orthodox Jews, among others, are commanded to follow certain precautions regarding diet, alcohol, hygiene, and other *health-related behaviors* that are known favorably to impact morbidity and mortality.

• The collective aspect of spiritual practices provides *social support*, which has been documented as a potent protective factor against illness.

• The *psychodynamics of religious beliefs and religious rites* can also promote health. For example, rituals such as prayer may trigger a myriad of emotions which, in turn, may lead to changes in health by positively impacting the immune and cardiovascular systems.

• The *psychodynamics of faith* can be indistinguishable from the placebo effect, if one expects God's blessings (or the nocebo or "negative placebo" effect, if one expects God's wrath and punishment!).[3]

- Experiencing the presence of a healer or healers may foster a sense of belonging or support, which research shows is healthful.
- Being the object of prayer or of laying on of hands or other ritualized activity may stimulate an endocrine or immune response facilitative of healing.
- The physical preparations for healing (e.g., preliminary feasts, meditation, abstentions of one sort or another) may themselves be promotive of health. [4]

These findings have been affirmed for *mental* health by NIH physician-researcher David B. Larson and Susan S. Larson. They surveyed twelve years of publication of the *American Journal of Psychiatry* and *Archives of General Psychiatry* and found that, when measuring participation in religious ceremony, social support, prayer, and relationship with God, 92 percent of the studies showed benefit for mental health, 4 percent were neutral, and 4 percent showed harm.[5] F. C. Craigie and his colleagues, in a 1990 review of ten years of publication of the *Journal of Family Practice*, found similar findings for *physical* health: 83 percent of the studies showed benefit, 17 percent were neutral, and none showed harm.[6]

There is evidence that the scientific and medical community may be slowly opening to the cumulative scientific evidence we have examined in this book. As an indicator, the newly established Office of Alternative Medicine of the National Institutes of Health directed its panel on Mind/Body Interventions to examine the evidence surrounding the effectiveness of prayer and spiritual healing.

Those who believe in prayer might pray for this process to continue.

Notes

AUTHOR'S NOTE

1. Clifton Wolters, trans., *The Cloud of Unknowing* (Baltimore: Penguin Books, 1961), 59.
2. Edmund Colledge and Bernard McGinn, trans., *Meister Eckhart* (New York: Paulist Press, 1981), 204–5.
3. Raymond B. Blakney, trans., *Meister Eckhart* (New York: Harper & Row, 1941), 243.

PREFACE

1. These studies are summarized in Appendix 1.
2. Many books have recently been published that describe these new developments. A splendid example is Willis W. Harman, *A Re-Examination of the Metaphysical Foundations of Modern Science* (Sausalito, CA: Institute of Noetic Sciences, 1991).

INTRODUCTION

1. Father Andrew Greeley, "Keeping the Faith: Americans Hold Fast to the Rock of Ages," *OMNI* 13:11 (August 1991): 6. See also Kenneth L. Woodward, *et al.*, "Talking to God," *Newsweek* (January 6, 1992): 38–44.
2. Stanley Krippner and Patrick Welch, *Spiritual Dimensions of Healing: From Native Shamanism to Contemporary Health Care* (New York: Irvington Publishers, 1992), 196.
3. Lawrence LeShan, *From Newton to ESP* (Wellingborough, Northamptonshire, England: Turnstone Press Limited, 1984), 172. Republished later as *The Science of the Paranormal: The Last Frontier* (Wellingborough, Northamptonshire, England: The Aquarian Press, 1987).
4. LeShan, *From Newton to ESP*, 174.
5. C. S. Lewis, *Letters to Malcolm: Chiefly on Prayer* (New York: Harcourt Brace Jovanovich, 1964), 28.
6. R. J. Foster, *Prayer: Finding the Heart's True Home* (San Francisco: HarperSanFrancisco, 1992), vii.
7. Ann Ulanov and Barry Ulanov, *Primary Speech: A Psychology of Prayer* (Atlanta: John Knox Press, 1982), vii.
8. Eugene C. Kreider, "Learning and Teaching Prayer," in Paul R. Sponheim, ed., *A Primer on Prayer* (Philadelphia: Fortress Press, 1988), 143.

9. Lewis, *Letters to Malcolm*, 63.

10. Kathleen Raine quoted in "Interview," *Gnosis* (Spring 1992): 52.

11. André Malraux, quoted in interview with Michel de Salzmann, *Parabola* 8, no. 1 (January 1983).

1. SAINTS AND SINNERS, HEALTH AND ILLNESS

1. Retold from John White, *The Meeting of Science and Spirit: Guidelines for a New Age* (New York: Paragon House, 1990), 100.

2. A famous cleric once said, "God is interested in a lot more things than theology." In view of the frequent illnesses demonstrated by the saints and mystics, we might add that he also seems interested in a lot more things than health.

3. Two superb accounts of the complex interplay of health and illness have recently appeared. Arthur Frank's *At the Will of the Body: Reflections on Illness* (Boston: Houghton Mifflin, 1991) is extraordinarily sensitive and wise. Frank, a professor of sociology, experienced a heart attack and cancer within two years and survived both. Kat Duff's *The Alchemy of Illness* (New York: Pantheon, 1993), describes her struggle with chronic fatigue syndrome. This insightful account is also a beautifully literary work.

4. It may be of interest at this point to note that Campbell died of cancer. See Stephen Larsen and Robin Larsen, *A Fire in the Mind: The Life of Joseph Campbell* (New York: Doubleday, 1991).

5. Michael Toms, *Interviews with Joseph Campbell*. New Dimensions Radio, 475 Gate Five Road, Suite 206, Sausalito, CA 94966.

6. Rainer Maria Rilke, *Letters to a Young Poet*, translated by M. D. Herter Norton (New York: W. W. Norton, 1934), 69–70.

7. Adapted from Natalie Goldberg, *Wild Mind: Living the Writer's Life* (New York: Bantam, 1990).

8. Retold from John White, *The Meeting of Science and Spirit: Guidelines for a New Age* (New York: Paragon House, 1990), 105.

9. Raymond B. Blakney, trans., *Meister Eckhart* (New York: Harper & Row, 1941), 249–50.

10. Clifton Wolters, trans., *The Cloud of Unknowing* (Baltimore: Penguin Books, 1961), 76.

11. "Higher health" is a theme running through my book *Beyond Illness: Discovering the Experience of Health* (Boston: Shambhala, 1984).

12. Quoted in "Sunbeams," *The Sun* 192 (November 1991): 40.

13. Quoted in Ernest Kurtz and Katherine Ketcham, *The Spirituality of Imperfection: Modern Wisdom from Classic Stories* (New York: Bantam, 1992), 221–22. Kurtz and Ketcham point out a little-known fact: the word *islam* means "submission." The story is retold from Idries Shah, *The Way of the Sufi* (New York: E. P. Dutton, 1968), 190.

14. Personal communication, April 1992, source anonymous.

15. Quoted in "Sunbeams," *The Sun* 198 (May 1992): 40.

16. Story related by Ananth Krishnan, Grand Blanc, Michigan, February 1991.

17. William Boyd, *The Spontaneous Regression of Cancer* (Springfield, IL: Charles C. Thomas, 1966), 5 and 89.

18. Boyd, *The Spontaneous Regression of Cancer*, 8–9.

19. T. C. Everson and W. H. Cole, *The Spontaneous Regression of Cancer* (Philadelphia: Saunders, 1966).

20. For a review of the shifting attitudes on this subject throughout our history, see Lawrence LeShan, *Cancer As a Turning Point* (New York: E. P. Dutton, 1989).

21. Yujiro Ikemi, Shunji Nakagawa, Tetsuya Nakagawa, and Mineyasu Sugita, "Psychosomatic Consideration on Cancer Patients Who Have Made a Narrow Escape from Death," *Dynamic Psychiatry* 31 (1975): 77–92.

22. Nikos Kazantzakis, *The Saviors of God*, translated by Kimon Friar (New York: Simon & Schuster, 1960), 128–29.

23. Manly P. Hall, quoted in Stephan A. Hoeller, "The Spirit in Health and Disease," *Gnosis* (Spring 1991): 8–9.

24. Lewis Thomas, quoted in Patricia Norris, "Self-Regulation Through Imagery," *ISSSEEM Newsletter* (The International Society for the Study of Subtle Energies and Energy Medicine) 3:2 (Summer 1992): 4–8.

25. Rachel Naomi Remen, "Your Emotions and Your Health," *Unity* 172, no. 10 (October 1992): 48–54.

26. James Hillman, interviewed by Sy Syfransky, "The Myths of Our Therapy Culture," *Yoga Journal* 104 (May/June 1992): 52 ff.

27. For a penetrating critique of this point of view, the writings of transpersonal psychologist Ken Wilber are indispensable. Particularly recommended is his poignant book about his wife's experience with cancer, *Grace and Grit* (Boston: Shambhala, 1991).

28. H. Morganstern, G. A. Gellert, S. D. Walter, A. M. Ostfeld, and B. S. Siegal, "The Impact of a Psychosocial Support Program on Survival with Breast Cancer: The Importance of Selection Bias in Program Evaluation," *Journal of Chronic Disease* 37: 273. See also G. A. Gellert, R. M. Maxwell, and B. S. Siegal, "Survival of Breast Cancer Patients Receiving Adjunctive Psychosocial Support Therapy: A 10-Year Follow-up Study," *Journal of Clinical Oncology* 2:1, 1993, 66–69.

29. Henry Dreher, "Behavioral Medicine's New Marketplace of Clinical Applications: A Report on a Conference," *Advances* 8, no. 2 (Spring 1992): 46–69.

30. Susan Ertz, quoted in "Sunbeams," *The Sun* 196 (March 1992): 40.

2. THE REACH OF THE MIND:
SETTING THE STAGE FOR PRAYER

1. I. Regardie, *The Philosopher's Stone* (St. Paul, MN: Llewellyn Publications, 1970), 90. Quoted in Randolph Severson, "The Alchemy of Dreamwork: Reflections on Freud and the Alchemical Tradition," *Dragonflies* (Spring 1979): 109.

2. P. B. Amar, ed., *Standards and Guidelines for Biofeedback Applications in Psychophysiological Self-Regulation*, Applications Standards Committee of the Association for Applied Psychophysiology and Biofeedback (Wheat Ridge, CO.: Association for Applied Psychophysiology and Biofeedback, 1992). See also R. Shellenberger, P. Amar, C. Schneider, and R. Steward, *Clinical Efficacy and Cost Effectiveness of Biofeedback Therapy* (Wheat Ridge, CO: Association for Applied Psychophysiology and Biofeedback, 1989).

3. Erwin Schrödinger, *What is Life? and Mind and Matter* (London: Cambridge University Press, 1969), 145.

4. Carl Sagan, quoted in *Brain/Mind Bulletin* 6:5 (February 16, 1981): 1.

5. C. Norman Shealy and Caroline M. Myss, *The Creation of Health: Merging Traditional Medicine with Intuitive Diagnosis* (Walpole, NH: Stillpoint, 1988).

6. Shealy and Myss, *The Creation of Health*, 73 ff.

7. The custom of snap diagnosis was engaged in by some of the greatest physicians of the day. These events have never been fully explained. They represent a kind of historical embarrassment for modern scientific medicine, which denies they are possible. They raise profound questions about how physicians arrive at diagnoses, and suggest that the process may not always be as rational as presumed.

8. F. H. Garrison, *History of Medicine*, 4th ed. (Philadelphia: W. B. Saunders, 1928), 757.

9. Dolores Krieger, *Foundations of Holistic Health: Nursing Practices* (Philadelphia: J. P. Lippincott, 1981). See also Dolores Krieger, *The Therapeutic Touch* (Englewood Cliffs, NJ: Prentice Hall, 1979). See also Dolores Krieger, *Accepting Your Power to Heal* (Santa Fe: Bear & Company Publishing, 1993).

10. Daniel P. Wirth, "The Effect of Non-contact Therapeutic Touch on the Healing of Full Thickness Dermal Wounds," *Subtle Energies* 1:1, 1–20.

    See also the pioneering work of Janet Quinn, "Therapeutic Touch as Energy Exchange: Testing the Theory," *Advances in Nursing Science* 6 (1984): 42–49, and Janet Quinn, *An Investigation of the Effects of Therapeutic Touch Done without Physical Contact on State Anxiety of Hospitalized Cardiovascular Patients*. Doctoral dissertation, New York University, 1982, University Microfilm #DA8226788.

11. For effect of Therapeutic Touch on hemoglobin levels, see D. Krieger, "Therapeutic Touch: The Imprimatur of Nursing," *American Journal of Nursing* 7 (1975): 784–867.

   For effect of Therapeutic Touch on healing of full-thickness skin wounds, see Wirth, "Unorthodox Healing."

   For effect of Therapeutic Touch on tension headache, see E. Keller and V. M. Bzkek, "Effects of Therapeutic Touch on Tension Headache Pain," *Nursing Research* (1986): 101–4.

   For effect of Therapeutic Touch on postoperative pain, see T. C. Meehan, *An Abstract of the Effect of Therapeutic Touch on the Experience of Acute Pain in Post-Operative Patients*, unpublished Ph.D. dissertation, New York University, 1985.

   For effect of Therapeutic Touch on anxiety, see P. Heidt, *An Investigation of the Effect of Therapeutic Touch on the Anxiety of Hospitalized Patients*, unpublished Ph.D. dissertation, New York University, 1979.

   See also Quinn, *An Investigation of the Effect of Therapeutic Touch without Physical Contact on State Anxiety of Hospitalized Cardiovascular Patients*; C. K. Ferguson, *Subjective Experience of Therapeutic Touch (SETTS): Psychometric Examination of an Instrument*, unpublished Ph.D. dissertation, University of Texas at Austin, 1986; R. B. Fedoruk, *Transfer of the Relaxation Response: Therapeutic Touch as a Method for the Reduction of Stress in Premature Neonates*, unpublished Ph.D. dissertation, University of Maryland, 1984; J. W. Collins, *The Effect of Non-Contact Therapeutic Touch on the Relaxation Response*, unpublished master's thesis, Vanderbilt University, 1983; G. L. Randolph, *The Differences in Psychological Response of Female College Students Exposed to Stressful Stimulus, When Simultaneously Treated by Either Therapeutic Touch or Casual Touch*, unpublished Ph.D. dissertation, New York University, 1979; and B. S. Parkes, *Therapeutic Touch as an Intervention to Reduce Anxiety in Elderly Hospitalized Patients*, unpublished Ph.D. dissertation, University of Texas at Austin, 1985.

12. Jeanne Achterberg, *Imagery in Healing* (Boston: New Science Library, 1986).

13. William G. Braud and Marilyn Schlitz, "A Method for the Objective Study of Transpersonal Imagery," *Journal of Scientific Exploration* 3, no. 1 (1989): 43–63.

14. Robert G. Jahn and Brenda J. Dunne, *Margins of Reality: The Role of Consciousness in the Physical World* (New York: Harcourt Brace Jovanovich, 1987).

15. Franz Hartmann, *Paracelsus: Life and Prophecies* (Blauvelt, NY: Steinerbooks, 1973), 133. See also Robert J. Sardello, "Samuel Hahnemann and the Alchemical Tradition," *Artifex* 10 (1992): 17–28.

16. Berthold E. Schwarz, "Possible Telesomatic Reactions," *The Journal of the Medical Society of New Jersey* 64, no.11: 600–603.

17. E. Gurney, F. W. H. Myers, and F. Podmore, *Phantasms of the Living* (London: Trübner, 1886), 188–89.

18. Louisa E. Rhine, "Psychological Processes in ESP Experiences. Part I. Waking Experiences," *Journal of Parapsychology* 29 (1962): 88–111.

19. J. H. Rush, "New Directions in Parapsychological Research," *Parapsychological Monographs No. 4* (New York: Parapsychology Foundation, 1964), 18–19.

20. T. Blaksley, "Impression," *Journal of the Society for Psychical Research* 5 (1892): 241.

21. One of the best analyses of these events is Ian Stevenson, *Telepathic Impressions: A Review of 35 New Cases* (Charlottesville: University Press of Virginia, 1970).

22. Schwarz, "Possible Telesomatic Reactions," 600–603.

23. Rhine, "Psychological Processes in ESP Experiences. Part I. Waking Experiences," 123–24.

24. Stevenson, *Telepathic Impressions*, 14–15.

25. Jean Lanier, "From Having a Mystical Experience to Becoming a Mystic—Reprint and Epilogue," *ReVision* 12, no. 1 (Summer 1989): 41–44.

26. Lanier, "From Having a Mystical Experience to Becoming a Mystic," 41.

27. Helen Tworkov, *Zen in America* (San Francisco: North Point Press, 1989), 225. For a brilliant discussion of the relationship between parapsychological experiences and spiritual growth, see Donald Evans, *Spirituality and Human Nature* (Albany, NY: State University of New York Press), 1993.

28. Ian Stevenson, *Telepathic Impressions*, 144.

3. PRAYER AND THE UNCONSCIOUS MIND

1. Retold from Larry Dossey, *Meaning & Medicine* (New York: Bantam, 1991), 29–30.

2. David Spiegel, "A Psychosocial Intervention and Survival Time of Patients with Metastatic Breast Cancer," *Advances* 7, no. 3 (Summer 1991): 10–19.

3. Spiegel, "A Psychosocial Intervention," 15.

4. For a review of the "side effects of positive thinking" and problems associated with the "force-feeding of hope," see Karen Ritchie, "Guilt and the Cancer Patient," *The Cancer Bulletin* (of the University of Texas M. D. Anderson Cancer Center, Houston, Texas) 43, no. 5 (1991): 430–32; and Ross E. Gray and Brian D. Doan, "Heroic Self-Healing and Cancer: Clinical Issues for the Health Professions," *Journal of Palliative Care* 6, no. 1 (1990): 32–41.

5. For a review of the role of the unconscious mind, see Daniel Goleman, *Vital Lies, Simple Truths: The Psychology of Self-Deception* (New York: Touchstone, 1985).

6. Thomas P. Hackett and Jerrold E. Rosenbaum, "Emotion, Psychiatric Disorders, and the Heart," in Eugene Braunwald, *Heart Disease: A Textbook of Cardiovascular Medicine* (Philadelphia: W. B. Saunders, 1980), 1923–43.

7. Alexander Leaf, "Preventive Medicine for Our Ailing Health Care System," *Journal of the American Medical Association* 269, no. 5 (February 3, 1993): 616–18.

8. Shelley E. Taylor, *Positive Illusions: Creative Self-Deception and the Healthy Mind* (New York: Basic Books, 1989).

9. Bruce Bower, "Anxiety Before Surgery May Prove Helpful," *Science News* 141 (June 20, 1992): 406–7.

10. ibid., 406-7

11. Jayne Gackenbach and Jane Bosveld, *Control Your Dreams* (New York: HarperPerennial, 1990), 108–9.

12. William G. Braud, "Consciousness Interactions with Remote Biological Systems: Anomalous Intentionality Effects," *Subtle Energies* (Journal of the International Society for the Study of Subtle Energies and Energy Medicine) 2, no. 1: 1–46.

13. See Brendan O'Regan, "Healing, Remission and Miracle Cures," *Institute of Noetic Sciences Special Report* (May 1987): 3–14.

14. Gary Snyder, "The Etiquette of Freedom," *Sierra* 74, no. 5 (September-October 1989): 75 ff. See also Haniel Long, *The Marvelous Adventure of Cabeza de Vaca* (Clear Lake, CA: The Dawn Horse Press), 1992.

15. Will Steger, "Six Across Antarctica," *National Geographic* 178:5 (November 1990): 67–93. A full-length account of the trek can be found in Will Steger and Jon Bowermaster, *Crossing Antarctica* (New York: Alfred A. Knopf, 1991).

16. Adapted from Gary Snyder, "The Etiquette of Freedom," *Sierra* 74, no. 5 (1989), 75 ff.

17. P. W. Bridgman, *The Way Things Are* (Cambridge: Harvard University Press, 1966), 154.

18. R. Davenport, *An Outline of Animal Development* (Reading, MA: Addison-Wesley, 1979), 353.

19. Richard J. Foster, *Prayer: Finding the Heart's True Home* (San Francisco: HarperSanFrancisco, 1992), 117.

20. Foster, *Prayer,* 117.

21. Gackenbach and Bosveld, *Control Your Dreams,* 190.

22. Gackenbach and Bosveld, *Control Your Dreams,* 190–91.

23. Gackenbach and Bosveld, *Control Your Dreams,* 195–96.

24. Gackenbach and Bosveld, *Control Your Dreams,* 197.

25. Sandra Ingerman, *Welcome Home: Life After Healing* (San Francisco: Harper-SanFrancisco, 1993). See also Sandra Ingerman, *Soul Retrieval: Mending the Fragmented Self* (San Francisco: HarperSanFrancisco, 1991).

26. "Letters: Readers' Tales of Trauma and Typewriters," *Brain/Mind Bulletin and Common Sense*, vol. 18, no. 7, April 1993, p. 8.

27. Jeanne Achterberg, *Imagery in Healing* (Boston: Shambhala, 1985).

28. Gackenbach and Bosveld, *Control Your Dreams*, 101.

29. Gackenbach and Bosveld, *Control Your Dreams*, 100–101.

30. L. L. Vasiliev, *Experiments in Distant Influence* (New York: E. P. Dutton, 1963), 84 ff.

31. Vasiliev, *Experiments in Distant Influence*, 92–93.

32. R. Desoille, "De quelque conditions auxquelles il faut satisfaire pour réussir des expériences de télepathie provoquée," *Revue Métapsychique*, no. 6 (1932). See Vasiliev, *Experiments in Distant Influence*, 95.

33. Sigmund Freud, "The Unconscious," in J. Strachey, ed. and trans., *The Standard Edition of the Complete Psychological Works of Sigmund Freud* (London: Hogarth Press, 1957; originally published in 1915), vol. 14, 159–215. Cited in Christine M. Comstock, "The Inner Self Helper and Concepts of Inner Guidance: Historical Antecedents, Its Role within Dissociation, and Clinical Utilization," *Dissociation* 4, no. 3 (September 1991): 170.

34. Comstock, "The Inner Self Helper," 170.

35. Montague Ullman and Stanley Krippner, with Alan Vaughan, *Dream Telepathy: Experiments in Nocturnal ESP*, 2d ed. (Jefferson, NC: McFarland, 1989), 111–12. See also Stanley Krippner and Patrick Welch, *Spiritual Dimensions of Healing* (New York: Irvington, 1992), 188–89.

36. Lawrence LeShan, *The Medium, the Mystic, and the Physicist* (New York: Viking, 1974), p. 125.

37. This complicates such experiments considerably, because the prayed-for group, *knowing* they are being prayed for, become more susceptible to the effects of suggestion—the placebo response.

38. Lawrence LeShan, *The Medium, the Mystic, and the Physicist* (New York: Viking, 1974), p. 120.

39. Quoted in "Sunbeams," *The Sun* 198 (May 1992): 40.

40. Gerhard Adler and Aniela Jaffé, eds., *Jung's Letters*, vol. 1 (Princeton: Princeton University Press, 1973), 377.

4. WHERE DO PRAYERS GO?

1. Nick Herbert, *Quantum Reality* (New York: Anchor Books, 1987), 214.

2. Herbert, *Quantum Reality*, 249. See also Amit Goswami, "The Idealistic Interpretation of Quantum Mechanics," *Physics Essays* 2, no. 4 (1989): 385–400.

Goswami is a theoretical physicist at the University of Oregon's Department of Physics and the Institute of Theoretical Science. This paper is an excellent explanation of why many theorists in physics regard mind as nonlocal—unbounded, unitary, and in some sense one.

3. Larry Dossey, *Recovering the Soul* (New York: Bantam, 1989).

4. See N. D. Mermin, *Physics Today* 38 (1985): 38, and Heinz R. Pagels, *The Cosmic Code* (New York: Simon and Schuster, 1982), 160–76.

5. Herbert, *Quantum Reality*, 249–50.

6. Kenneth Woodward, et al., "Talking to God," *Newsweek* (January 6, 1992): 38–44.

7. Woodward, et al., "Talking to God," 44.

5. HOW TO PRAY AND WHAT TO PRAY *FOR*

1. See Jean Gill, *Pray as You Can: Discovering Your Own Prayer Ways* (Notre Dame, IN: Ave Maria Press, 1989). Quoted also in Richard J. Foster, *Prayer: Finding the Heart's True Home* (San Francisco: HarperSanFrancisco, 1992), 1.

2. For a summary of the religious words and phrases used in various Western traditions, which Benson found effective, see Herbert Benson, M.D., *Beyond the Relaxation Response* (New York: Times Books, 1984). See also Aldous Huxley, "Ritual, Symbol, Sacrament" and "Spiritual Exercises," *The Perennial Philosophy* (New York: Harper & Row, 1944), 262–92.

3. Stephen Keisling and T George Harris, "The Prayer War," *Psychology Today*, October 1989, pp. 65 ff.

4. Joan Borysenko, *Fire in the Soul: A New Psychology of Spiritual Optimism* (New York: Warner Books, 1993), 161–88.

5. Jon Kabat-Zinn, *Full Catastrophe Living: Using the Wisdom of Your Body and Mind to Face Stress, Pain and Illness* (New York: Delacorte Press, 1990).

6. See Chester P. Michael and Marie C. Norriscy, "Discovering Your Personality Type," in *Prayer and Temperament: Different Prayer Forms for Different Personality Types* (Charlottesville, VA: The Open Door, 1984), 121–26.

7. For one of the best descriptions of Jung's psychology written for laypeople, see Laurens van der Post, *Jung and the Story of Our Time* (New York: Vintage/Random House, 1977).

8. June Singer, *Boundaries of the Soul: The Practice of Jung's Psychology* (New York: Anchor/Doubleday, 1972), 184.

9. Singer, *Boundaries of the Soul*, 184–85.

10. Singer, *Boundaries of the Soul*, 186–87.

11. Aldous Huxley, *The Perennial Philosophy* (New York: Harper & Row, 1944), 225–26.

12. Chester P. Michael and Marie C. Norrisey, *Prayer and Temperament: Different Prayer Forms for Different Personality Types* (Charlottesville, VA: The Open Door, 1984), 126.

13. Evelyn Underhill, *Mysticism* (New York: E. P. Dutton, 1961).

14. Richard Jerome, "Born Shy," *The Sciences* (September/October 1991): 6.

15. Spindrift may be contacted at Spindrift, Inc., P.O. Box 3995, Salem, OR 97302–0995.

16. Robert Owen, *Qualitative Research: The Early Years* (Salem, OR: Grayhaven Books, 1988), 22–23.

17. Owen, *Qualitative Research*, 89.

18. Ann and Barry Ulanov, *Primary Speech: A Psychology of Prayer* (Atlanta: John Knox Press, 1982), 102–3.

19. Dennis Gersten, M.D., Interview with Janet Quinn, R.N., Ph.D., "AIDS, Hope and Healing," Part II, *Atlantis: The Imagery Newsletter* (February 1992): 3 ff.

20. William G. Braud, "The Influence of Consciousness in the Physical World: A Psychologist's View," paper presented to the Second International Symposium "Science and Consciousness," Athens, Greece, January 3–7, 1992.

21. William G. Braud, "Human Interconnectedness: Research Indications," *ReVision* 14, no.3 (Winter 1992): 140–48.

22. Braud, "Human Interconnectedness," 2.

23. Jeanne Achterberg, *Imagery in Healing* (Boston: Shambhala, 1985).

24. G. Porter and Patricia Norris, *Why Me?* (Walpole, NH: Stillpoint, 1986), 94.

25. This refers to the work of Dr. Howard Hall of Pennsylvania State University. See Steven Locke and Daniel Colligan, *The Healer Within* (New York: E. P. Dutton, 1986), 187–88.

26. Jeanne Achterberg and G. Frank Lawlis, *Imagery and Disease* (Champaign, IL: Institute for Personality and Ability Testing, 1984). See also Jeanne Achterberg, *Imagery in Healing: Shamanism and Modern Medicine* (Boston: Shambhala/New Science Library, 1985).

27. Mark S. Rider and Jeanne Achterberg, "Effect of Music-Associated Imagery on Neutrophils and Lymphocytes," *Biofeedback and Self-Regulation* 14, no.3 (1989): 247–57. A possible explanation why white blood cells seem usually to decrease and not increase in experimental situations such as this is that they may move outside the bloodstream into body tissues as part of their natural mission of surveillance, thereby becoming unavailable for counting when a blood sample is drawn. This suggests a healthy response to mental imagery, not an unhealthy one, as might be suggested by a "falling" white blood cell count. See C. W. Smith, J. Schneider, C. Minning, and S. Whitcher, *Imagery and Neutrophil Function Studies: A Preliminary Report*, unpublished manuscript, Michigan State University, 1983.

28. G. Richard Smith, et al., "Psychological Modulation of the Human Immune System Response to Varicella Zoster," *Archives of Internal Medicine* 145 (1985): 2110–12.

29. In addition to the works of Achterberg and Lawlis cited above, the following works of Sheikh are valuable references to the excellent work in this field: Anees A. Sheikh, ed., *Imagery: Current Theory, Research and Application* (New York: Wiley, 1983); *Imagination and Healing* (Farmingdale, NY: Baywood, 1984); *Anthology of Imagery Techniques* (Milwaukee: American Imagery Institute, 1986); Anees A. Sheikh and J. T. Shaffer, eds., *The Potential of Fantasy and Imagination* (New York: Brandon House, 1979); Anees A. Sheikh and Katharina S. Sheikh, eds., *Eastern and Western Approaches to Healing: Ancient Wisdom and Modern Knowledge* (New York: Wiley, 1989); and Anees A. Sheikh and Katharina S. Sheikh, eds., *Death Imagery* (Milwaukee: American Imagery Institute, 1991).

30. Chuang Tzu, *Chuang Tzu: Basic Writings*, Burton Watson, trans. (New York: Columbia University Press, 1964), quoted in *Parabola* 8, no. 3 (August 1983): 70.

31. Clifton Wolters, trans., *The Cloud of Unknowing and Other Works* (Harmondsworth, England: Penguin Books, 1964), cited in *Parabola* 8, no. 3 (August 1983): 64.

32. Joan Borysenko, *Guilt Is the Teacher, Love Is the Lesson* (New York: Warner Books, 1990), 181–82.

6. LOVE AND HEALING

1. H. Medalie and U. Goldbourt, "Angina Pectoris Among 10,000 Men II: Psychosocial and Other Risk Factors as Evidenced by a Multivariate Analysis of Five-year Incidence Study," *American Journal of Medicine* 60 (1976): 910–21.

2. Joan Borysenko, "Healing Motives: An Interview with David McClelland," *Advances* 2 (1985): 29–41.

3. Steven Locke and Douglas Colligan, *The Healer Within: The New Medicine of Mind and Body* (New York: E. P. Dutton, 1986), 211.

4. Quoted in Robert G. Jahn and Brenda J. Dunne, *Margins of Reality: The Role of Consciousness in the Physical World* (New York: Harcourt Brace Jovanovich, 1987), 343.

5. Lawrence LeShan, *The Medium, the Mystic, and the Physicist* (New York: Viking, 1974), 107.

6. Joseph Banks Rhine and Sara R. Feather, "The Study of Cases of 'Psi-trailing' in Animals," *The Journal of Parapsychology* 26, no. 1 (March 1962): 1–21.

7. Vida Adamoli, "Incredible Animals," *Good Housekeeping* (April 1991): 116. From Vida Adamoli, *The Dog that Drove Home, the Snake-Eating Mouse, and Other Exotic Tales from the Animal Kingdom* (New York: St. Martin's Press, 1991).

8. The actual details of these machines and how they operate is not our concern here; they have been described in Robert G. Jahn and Brenda J. Dunne, *Margins of Reality* (New York: Harcourt Brace Jovanovich, 1987).

9. Stanley Krippner, "The Synergy Project: A Worthy Enterprise in Need of Clarification," *ICIS Forum* 22, no. 2 (April 1992): 9–10.

10. Carl G. Jung, *Memories, Dreams, Reflections*, edited by Aniela Jaffé, translated by Richard and Clara Winston (New York: Vintage, 1965), 354.

11. Jung, *Memories, Dreams, Reflections*, 353.

12. Jung, *Memories, Dreams, Reflections*, 353.

7. TIME-DISPLACED PRAYER: WHEN PRAYERS ARE ANSWERED BEFORE THEY ARE MADE

1. Hans Eysenk and Carl Sargent, *Explaining the Unexplained* (London: Weidenfeld and Nicolson, 1982), 39.

2. Ray Hyman, quoted in Jeremy W. Hayward, *Shifting Worlds, Changing Minds* (Boston: Shambhala, 1987), 172.

3. Dean Radin and Roger Nelson, "Consciousness-Related Effects in Random Physical Systems," *Foundations of Physics* 19 (1989): 1499–1514.

4. William G. Braud and Marilyn J. Schlitz, "Time-Displaced Effects?" in "Consciousness Interactions with Remote Biological Systems: Anomalous Intentionality Effects," *Subtle Energies* 2, no. 1 (1992): 1–46. See H. Schmidt, "PK Effect on Pre-recorded Targets," *Journal of the American Society for Psychical Research* 70 (1976): 267–91; H. Schmidt, "Can an Effect Precede Its Cause?" *Foundations of Physics* 8 (1981): 463–80; H. Schmidt, "Addition Effect for PK on Pre-recorded Targets," *Journal of Parapsychology* 49 (1985): 229–44.

5. H. Schmidt, "Superposition of PK Effects by Man and Dog," in *Research in Parapsychology 1983*, edited by R. White and R. Broughton (Metuchen, NJ: Scarecrow Press, 1984), 96–98. See also H. Schmidt, "Human PK Effort on Pre-recorded Random Events Previously Observed by Goldfish," in *Research in Parapsychology 1985*, edited by D. Weiner and D. Radin (Metuchen, NJ: Scarecrow Press, 1986), 18–21; and H. Schmidt, "The Strange Properties of Psychokinesis," *Journal of Scientific Exploration* 1, no. 2 (1987): 103–18.

6. W. G. Braud, G. Davis, and R. Wood, "Experiments with Matthew Manning," *Journal of the Society for Psychical Research* 50, no. 782 (1979): 199–223.

7. T. R. Harrison, "The Value and Limitation of Laboratory Tests in Clinical Medicine," *Journal of the Medical Association of Alabama* 12 (1944): 381–84, quoted in Stanley Joel Reiser, M.D., "The Era of the Patient," *Journal of the American Medical Association* 269, no. 8 (February 24, 1993): 1012–17.

8. Jeanne Achterberg, personal communication to the author, February 1992.

9. Ann and Barry Ulanov, *Primary Speech: A Psychology of Prayer* (Atlanta: John Knox Press, 1982), 103–4.

10. Nick Herbert, *Quantum Reality* (Garden City, NY: Anchor Press/Doubleday, 1987), 164–66.

11. Herbert, *Quantum Reality*, 166–67.

12. C. S. Lewis, *Miracles* (New York: Collier/Macmillan, 1960), 179.

13. For further discussion, see Joan Borysenko's "Why Bad Things Happen" in *Fire in the Soul: A New Psychology of Spiritual Optimism* (New York: Warner, 1933), 15–34.

8. YOUR DOCTOR'S BELIEFS AND WHY THEY MATTER

1. H. Rehder, "Wunderheilungen: Ein Experiment," *Hippokrates* 26 (1955): 577–80, cited in Jerry Solfvin, "Mental Healing," in *Advances in Parapsychological Research, Volume 4*, edited by Stanley Krippner (Jefferson, NC: McFarland and Company, 1984), 52.

2. W. M. Toone, "Effects of Vitamin E: Good and Bad," *New England Journal of Medicine* 289 (1973): 689–98.

3. T. W. Anderson, "Vitamin E in Angina Pectoris," *Canadian Medical Association Journal* 110 (1974): 401-6; and R. Gillian, B. Mondell, and J. R. Warbasse, "Quantitative Evaluation of Vitamin E in the Treatment of Angina Pectoris," *American Heart Journal* 93 (1977): 444–49.

4. E. H. Uhlenhuth, A. Cantor, J. O. Neustadt, and H. E. Payson, "The Symptomatic Relief of Anxiety with Meprobamate, Phenobarbital and Placebo," *American Journal of Psychiatry* 115 (1959): 905–10.

5. E. H. Uhlenhuth, K. Rickels, S. Fisher, L. C. Park, R. S. Lipman, and J. Mock, "Drug, Doctor's Verbal Attitude and Clinical Setting in the Symptomatic Response to Pharmacotherapy," *Psychopharmacologia* 9 (1966): 392–418.

6. J. Solfvin, "Mental Healing," in *Advances in Parapsychological Research, Volume 4*, edited by Stanley Krippner (Jefferson, NC: McFarland and Company, 1984), 55–56. See also: D. M. Engelhardt and R. Margolis, "Drug Identity, Doctor Conviction and Outcome," in H. Brill, ed., *Proceedings of the Fifth International Congress of Neuropsychopharmacology* (Amsterdam: Excerpta Medica Foundation, 1967); P. E. Feldman, "The Personal Element in Psychiatric Research," *American Journal of Psychiatry* 113 (1956): 52–54; C. R. B. Joyce, "Differences Between Physicians as Revealed by Clinical Trials," *Proceedings of the Royal Society of Medicine* 55 (1962): 776; W. Modell and R. W. Houde, "Factors Influencing the Clinical Evaluation of Drugs: With Special Reference to the Double-Blind Technique," *Journal of the American Medical Association* 167 (1958): 2190–99; M. Williams and T. F. McGee, "The Bias of the

Drug Administration in Judgments of the Effects of Psychopharmacological Agents," *Journal of Nervous and Mental Disease* 135 (1962): 569–73.

7. Jule Eisenbud, *Psi and Psychoanalysis* (New York: Grune & Stratton, 1970).

8. Martin Gardner, "Water With Memory? The Dilution Affair," in *The Hundredth Monkey*, edited by Kendrick Frazier (Buffalo, NY: Prometheus Books, 1991), 364.

9. Donald O. Hebb, *Organization of Behavior: A Neuropsychological Theory* (New York: Wiley, 1949), xiii.

10. Barry L. Beyerstein, "The Brain and Consciousness: Implications for Psi Phenomena," in Frazier, *The Hundredth Monkey*, 44.

11. Marcello Truzzi, professor of sociology at Eastern Michigan University at Ypsilanti, Michigan, and director of the Center for Scientific Anomalies Research at Ann Arbor, Michigan, has commented on the psychology of scientists. "Many studies in the psychology of science," he says, ". . . indicate that scientists are at least as dogmatic and authoritarian, at least as foolish and illogical as everybody else, including when they do science." Marcello Truzzi, in Simona Solovey, "Reflections on the Reception of Unconventional Claims in Science," *Frontier Perspectives* (publication of The Center for Frontier Sciences at Temple University) 1, no. 2 (Fall/Winter 1990): 12 ff.

12. Doug Boyd, *Rolling Thunder* (New York: Random House, 1974).

9. WHEN PRAYER HURTS: AN INQUIRY
INTO "BLACK PRAYER"

1. Sam Vincent Meddis, "Noriega Jurors Will Be Quizzed About Prayers," *USA Today* (May 28, 1992): 3A.

2. John Carey, "Wrath, Sanctity, and Power: The Cranky Saints of Ireland," *Gnosis*, no. 24, Summer 1992, 43–47.

3. Sir James Frazer, *The Golden Bough: A Study in Magic and Religion* (New York: Macmillan, 1922), 13–14.

4. E. A. Rauscher and B. A. Rubik, "Effects of Motility Behavior and Growth Rate of *Salmonella typhimurium* in the presence of Olga Worrall," in *Research in Parapsychology* (Metuchen, NJ, and London: Scarecrow Press, 1980), 140–42. See also E. A. Rauscher and B. A. Rubik, "Human Volitional Effects on a Model Bacterial System," *Psi Research* 2:1 (1983): 38.

5. Citations of Grad's experiments are provided in Appendix 1.

6. Personal communication to the author, June 1992.

7. C. B. Nash, "Test of Psychokinetic Control of Bacterial Mutation," *Journal of the American Society for Psychical Research* 78, no. 2 (1984): 145–52. See also C. B. Nash, "Psychokinetic Control of Bacterial Growth," *Journal of the American Society for Psychical Research* 51 (1982): 217–21.

8. J. Barry, "General and Comparative Study of the Psychokinetic Effect on a Fungus Culture," *Journal of Parapsychology* 32 (1968): 237–43.

9. Daniel J. Benor, "Survey of Spiritual Healing Research," *Complementary Medical Research* 4:3 (September 1990): 10–11.

10. Luther Burbank quoted in Robert Peel, *The Years of Authority* (New York: Holt, Rinehart and Winston, 1977), p. 348.

11. C. Flammarion, *L'Inconnu et les problemes psychiques* (Paris: 1900); reported in L. L. Vasiliev, *Experiments in Distant Influence* (New York: E. P. Dutton, 1976), 108–27 and 209–14.

12. Vasiliev, *Experiments in Distant Influence*, 108.

13. Vasiliev, *Experiments in Distant Influence*, 109.

14. It is not difficult to see why these questions cause considerable intellectual indigestion among anthropologists and many other types of scholars. Distant hexing suggests "action at a distance"—but distant, unmediated events are prohibited in principle because there is no scientific explanation for how they might occur. Since they *can't* occur, many scholars insist that they *don't* occur. Thus evidence to the contrary is often dismissed without a fair hearing.

15. Because this negative hexing lore is *so* spectacular, it is easy to lose sight of the more common positive, benevolent uses of shamanism. These are exemplified in a remarkable book, *Soul Retrieval*, by a modern psychologist and shaman Sandra Ingerman, who employs the traditional shamanic journey to bring about extraordinary physical and psychological healings in her patients. See Sandra Ingerman, *Soul Retrieval* (San Francisco: HarperSanFrancisco, 1991).

16. Walter Cannon, "'Voodoo' Death," *American Anthropologist* 44 (1942): 169–81.

17. See "Voodoo Death: The 'No Exit' Syndrome," in Larry Dossey, *Meaning & Medicine* (New York: Bantam, 1991), 57–61. See also Joan Halifax-Grof, "Hex Death," in Allan Angoff and Diana Barth, eds., *Parapsychology and Anthropology*, proceedings of an international conference held in London, England, August 29–31, 1973 (Parapsychology Foundation, 1974), 59–79; and J. K. Boitnott, "Clinicopathological Conference: Case Presentation," *Bulletin of Johns Hopkins Hospital*, no. 120 (1967): 186–87.

18. Holger Kalweit, *Shamans, Healers, and Medicine Men* (Boston: Shambhala, 1992).

19. Neal Claremon, *Coyote On a Wounded Planet: Ways of Knowing, Healing, and Connecting*, unpublished manuscript.

20. Abridged from Kalweit, *Shamans, Healers, and Medicine Men*, 184.

21. Abridged from Kalweit, *Shamans, Healers, and Medicine Men*, 184–85. Kalweit cites R. M. Berndt, "Wuradjeri Magic and 'Clever Men,'" *Oceania* 17 (1946–47): 327–65, and 18 (1947–48): 60–86.

22. Halifax-Grof, "Hex Death," 68.

23. Halifax-Grof, "Hex Death," 76.

24. Max Freedom Long, *The Secret Science Behind Miracles: Unveiling the Huna Tradition of the Ancient Polynesians* (Marina Del Rey, CA: DeVorss & Company, 1976).

25. Long, *The Secret Science Behind Miracles*, 1.

26. Long, *The Secret Science Behind Miracles*, 188–89.

27. See Goethe: "Two souls, alas, do dwell within my breast."

28. Long, *The Secret Science Behind Miracles*, 81.

29. Long, *The Secret Science Behind Miracles*, 279.

30. Long, *The Secret Science Behind Miracles*, 87.

31. The resemblance of these symptoms to Guillain-Barré syndrome, a neurological disease, is striking. The cause of this illness is unknown. This raises interesting questions: Could modern "diseases of unknown origin" sometimes be caused nonlocally by distant malevolent influences that escape detection? Unless we expand our worldview in modern medicine at least to *allow* for this possibility, we may never know.

32. Nick Herbert, *Quantum Reality* (New York: Anchor Books, 1987), 214.

33. Daniel J. Benor, "Research in Psychic Healing," in Betty Shapin and Lisette Coly, eds., *Current Trends in Psi Research*, proceedings of an international conference in New Orleans, Louisiana, 1984 (New York: Parapsychological Foundation, 1986), 96–119.

34. B. Onetto and G. H. Elguin, "Psychokinesis in Experimental Tumorogenesis" (Abstract), *Journal of Parapsychology* 30 (1966): 220.

10. GOD IN THE LABORATORY

1. Jacob Needleman, *A Sense of the Cosmos* (New York: E. P. Dutton, 1977).

2. Willis W. Harman, *A Re-Examination of the Metaphysical Foundations of Modern Science* (Sausalito, CA: Institute of Noetic Sciences, 1991), 71.

3. Robert G. Jahn and Brenda J. Dunne, *Margins of Reality: The Role of Consciousness in the Physical World* (New York: Harcourt Brace Jovanovich, 1987), 329–30.

4. *Webster's New World Dictionary*, Second College Edition, David B. Guralnik, Editor in Chief (New York: Prentice Hall, 1984), 1087.

5. For overviews of this field written for laypeople, see Harris Dienstfrey, *Where the Mind Meets the Body* (New York: HarperCollins, 1991), and Steven Locke, M.D., and Douglas Colligan, *The Healer Within: The New Science of Mind and Body* (New York: E. P. Dutton, 1986).

6. In medicine a substance that has no known biological effect but which causes harm to a patient is called a *nocebo*, as opposed to a *placebo*, which is beneficial.

11. PRAYER AND HEALING:
REVIEWING THE RESEARCH

1. Francis Galton, "Statistical Inquiries into the Efficacy of Prayer," *Fortnightly Review* 12 (1872): 125–35. Extracts of Galton's paper can be found in "Does Prayer Preserve?" *Archives of Internal Medicine* 125 (April 1970): 580–87.

2. "Eminent" persons were those distinguished enough to have had their lives recorded in a "biographical dictionary." Clergy eminent in their profession would presumably have been prayed for more than those of lesser notoriety.

3. John Polkinghorne, *Science and Providence: God's Interaction with the World* (Boston: New Science Library, 1989), 75.

4. Galton, "Statistical Inquiries," in *Archives of Internal Medicine*, 587.

5. For a description of Sheldrake's theories, see Rupert Sheldrake, *A New Science of Life: The Hypothesis of Formative Causation*, new ed. (London: Anthony Blond, 1982) and Rupert Sheldrake, *The Presence of the Past: Morphic Resonance and the Habits of Nature* (New York: New York Times Books, 1988).

6. William R. Parker and Elaine St. Johns, *Prayer Can Change Your Life* (New York: Prentice Hall Press, 1957).

7. William R. Parker and Elaine St. Johns, *Prayer Can Change Your Life* (New York: Prentice Hall Press, 1986 edition), p. ix.

8. P. J. Collipp, "The Efficacy of Prayer: A Triple Blind Study," *Medical Times* 97, no. 5 (1969): 201–4.

9. Benor has surveyed 131 controlled studies of spiritual healing published in the English literature, of which 56 showed statistically significant results. See Daniel J. Benor, "Survey of Spiritual Healing Research," *Complementary Medical Research* 4, no. 3 (September 1990): 9–33. This information is available in Appendix 1.

10. C. R. B. Joyce and R. M C. Welldon, "The Objective Efficacy of Prayer: A Double Blind Clinical Trial," *Journal of Chronic Disease* 18 (1965): 367–77.

11. Sir John Eccles, "The Human Person in Its Two-way Relationship to the Brain," in J. D. Morris, W. G. Roll, and R. L. Morris, eds., *Research in Parapsychology 1976* (Metuchen, NJ: Scarecrow Press, 1977), 251–62.

12. William G. Braud, "Distant Mental Influence of Rate of Hemolysis of Human Red Blood Cells," *Journal of the American Society for Psychical Research* 84, no. 1 (January 1990): 1–24.

13. Howard Wolinsky, "Prayers Do Aid Sick, Study Finds," *Chicago Sun-Times* (January 26, 1986): 30. Byrd's original study is published in Randolph C. Byrd, "Positive Therapeutic Effects of Intercessory Prayer in a Coronary Care Unit Population," *Southern Medical Journal* 81:7 (July 1988): 826–29.

14. Wolinsky, "Prayers Do Aid Sick, Study Finds," 30.

15. C. S. Lewis, *Letters to Malcolm: Chiefly on Prayer* (New York: Harcourt Brace Jovanovich, 1964), 18.

16. Thomas P. Hackett, *et al.*, "The Coronary Care Unit: An Appraisal of Its Psychological Hazards," *New England Journal of Medicine* 279 (1968): 1365. See also Thomas P. Hackett and Jerrold F. Rosenbaum, "Emotion, Psychiatric Disorders, and the Heart," in Eugene Braunwald, ed., *Heart Disease: A Textbook of Cardiovascular Medicine* (Philadelphia: W. B. Saunders, 1980), 1923–43.

17. Gary P. Posner, "God in the CCU?" *Free Inquiry* (Spring 1990): 44–45.

18. Daniel J. Benor, "Survey of Spiritual Healing Research," *Complementary Medical Research* 4, no. 1 (September 1990): 9–33.

19. J. Barry, "General and Comparative Study of the Psychokinetic Effect on a Fungus Culture," *Journal of Parapsychology* 32 (1968): 237–43.

20. W. Tedder and M. Monty, "Exploration of Long-distance PK: A Conceptual Replication of the Influence on a Biological System," *Research in Parapsychology 1980* (1981): 90–93.

21. C. B. Nash, "Psychokinetic Control of Bacterial Growth," *Journal of the American Society for Psychical Research* 51 (1982): 217–21.

22. B. Grad, "A Telekinetic Effect on Plant Growth: III. Stimulating and Inhibiting Effects." Research brief presented to the *Seventh Annual Convention of the Parapsychological Association*, Oxford University, 1964.

23. C. B. Nash, "Test of Psychokinetic Control of Bacterial Mutation," *Journal of the American Society for Psychical Research* 78, no. 2, (1984): 145–52.

24. Tim Friend, "Human Genes Can Mutate to Correct Defects," *USA Today* (February 18, 1993).

25. W. G. Braud, G. Davis, and R. Wood, "Experiments with Matthew Manning," *Journal of the American Society for Psychical Research* 50, no. 782 (1979): 199–223.

26. (a) N. Richmond, "Two Series of PK Tests on Paramecia," *Journal of the American Society for Psychical Research* 36 (1952): 577–78; (b) C. M. Pleass and N. D. Dey, "Using the Doppler Effect to Study Behavioral Responses of Motile Algae to Psi Stimulus," *Parapsychological Association Presented Papers* (1985): 373–405; (c) L. Metta, "Psychokinesis on Lepidopterous Larvae," *Journal of Parapsychology* 36 (1972): 213–21.

27. B. Grad, "Some Biological Effects of Laying-on of Hands: A Review of Experiments with Animals and Plants," *Journal of the American Society for Psychical Research* 59 (1965): 95–127.

28. B. Grad, R. J. Cadoret, and G. I. Paul, "The Influence of an Unorthodox Method of Treatment on Wound Healing in Mice," *International Journal of Parapsychology* 3 (1961): 5–24. See also B. Grad, "Some Biological Effects of

Laying-on of Hands: A Review of Experiments with Animals and Plants," *Journal of the American Society for Psychical Research* 59 (1965): 95–127; and B. Grad, "The 'Laying on of Hands' Implications for Psychotherapy, Gentling and the Placebo Effect," *Journal of the Society for Psychical Research* 61, no. 4 (1967): 286–305.

29. Grad, *et al.*, "The Influence of an Unorthodox Method"; Grad, "Some Biological Effects"; and Grad, "The 'Laying on of Hands.'"

30. Grad, *et al.*, "The Influence of an Unorthodox Method"; Grad, "Some Biological Effects"; and Grad, "The 'Laying on of Hands.'"

31. (a) G. K. Watkins and A. M. Watkins, "Possible PK Influence on the Resuscitation of Anesthetized Mice," *Journal of Parapsychology* 35, no. 4 (1971): 257–72; (b) G. K. Watkins, A. M. Watkins, and R. A. Wells, "Further Studies on the Resuscitation of Anesthetized Mice," *Research in Parapsychology 1972* (1973):157–59; (c) R. Wells and J. Klein, "A Replication of a 'Psychic Healing' Paradigm," *Journal of Parapsychology* 36 (1972): 144–47; (d) R. Wells and G. Watkins, "Linger Effects in Several PK Experiments," *Research in Parapsychology 1974* (1975): 143–47.

32. G. F. Solfvin, "Psi Expectancy Effects in Psychic Healing Studies with Malarial Mice," *European Journal of Parapsychology* 4, no. 2 (1982): 160–97.

12. WHAT IS HEALING?

1. Daniel J. Benor, "Believe It and You'll Be It: Visualization in Psychic Healing," *Psi Research* (March 1985): 42–43.

2. Lawrence LeShan, quoted in Benor, "Believe It and You'll Be It," 21–56.

3. Benor, "Believe It and You'll Be It," 36.

4. William G. Braud, "Healing Analog Research and Human Connectedness," paper presented at the Annual Meeting of the Society for the Scientific Study of Religion and the Religious Research Association, Virginia Beach, Virginia, November 9–11, 1990.

5. M. A. Persinger, "ELF Field Mediation in Spontaneous Psi Events: Direct Information Transfer or Conditioned Elicitation?" in Charles Tart, Harold Puthoff, and Russell Targ, eds., *Mind at Large* (New York: Praeger, 1979), 191–204.

6. Braud, "Healing Analog Research and Human Connectedness," 12.

7. R. G. Jahn, B. J. Dunne, and R. D. Nelson, "Engineering Anomalies Research," *Journal of Scientific Exploration* 1, no. 1 (1987): 21–50.

8. William G. Braud, "Using Living Targets in Psi Research," *Parapsychology Review* 20, no. 6 (1989): 1–4.

9. Daniel J. Benor, "A Psychiatrist Examines Fears of Healing," in *Newsletter* of the Consciousness Research and Training Project, Inc., edited by Joyce

Goodrich, Ph.D., 15, no. 1 (August 1991): 5–16. Address of Consciousness Research and Training Project, Inc.: 3215 East 68th Street, Box 9G, New York, NY 10021. The quotes from Benor in the rest of the chapter are from this source.

10. C.S. Lewis, *The Problem of Pain* (London: William Collins and Sons, 1977), p. 4

AFTERWORD

1. Pupul Jayakar, *Krishnamurti: A Biography* (San Francisco: Harper & Row, 1986), 485–86.

APPENDIX 1. CONTROLLED EXPERIMENTAL
TRIALS OF HEALING

1. Daniel J. Benor, "Survey of Spiritual Healing Research," *Complementary Medical Research* 4:1, September 1990, pp. 9–33; and Daniel J. Benor, *Healing Research* (Munich: Helix Verlag GmbH, 1993).

APPENDIX 2. SPONTANEOUS REGRESSION
OF CANCER

1. Yujiro Ikemi, Shunji Nakagawa, Tetsuya Nakagawa, and Mineyasu Sugita, "Psychosomatic Consideration on Cancer Patients Who Have Made a Narrow Escape from Death," *Dynamic Psychiatry* 31 (1975): 77–92.

APPENDIX 3. HOW GOOD IS THE EVIDENCE?
PRAYER, MEDITATION, AND PARAPSYCHOLOGY

1. D. Druckman and R. A. Bjork, eds., *In the Mind's Eye: Enhancing Human Performance* (Washington, D.C.: National Academy Press, 1991); D. Druckman and J. A. Swets, eds., *Enhancing Human Performance: Issues, Theories, and Techniques* (Washington, D.C.: National Academy Press, 1988).

2. Druckman and Bjork, *In the Mind's Eye*, 122.

3. D. S. Holmes, "Meditation and Somatic Arousal Reduction: A Review of the Experimental Evidence," *American Psychologist* 39, no. 1 (1984): 1–10.

4. J. Brener and S. R. Connally, "Meditation: Rationales, Experimental Effects, and Methodological Issues." Paper prepared for the U. S. Army Research Institute for the Behavioral and Social Sciences, European Division. Department of Psychology, University of Hull, London, England, 1986.

5. For an excellent summary of the techniques of meta-analysis applied to several parapsychological databases, see Jessica Utts, "Replication and Meta-analysis in Parapsychology," *Statistical Science* 6, no. 4 (1991): 363–403.

6. M. C. Dillbeck and D. W. Orme-Johnson, "Physiological Differences Between Transcendental Meditation and Rest," *American Psychologist* 42 (1987): 879–81. See also: C. N. Alexander, M. V. Rainforth, and P. Gelderloos,

"Transcendental Meditation, Self Actualization, and Psychological Health: A Conceptual Overview and Statistical Meta-analysis," *Journal of Social Behavior and Personality* 6, no. 5: 189–247.

7. K. R. Eppley, A. I. Abrams, and J. Shear, "Differential Effects of Relaxation Technique on Trait Anxiety: A Meta-analysis," *Journal of Clinical Psychology* 45, no. 6 (1989): 957–74.

8. Dillbeck and Orme-Johnson, "Physiological Differences Between Transcendental Meditation and Rest," 879–81. Also: Alexander, Rainforth, and Gelderloos, "Transcendental Meditation, Self Actualization, and Psychological Health," 189–247.

9. The data show that the TM-trained body operates at a lower baseline level of activity and has more adaptive reserves; hence the meditator may respond more powerfully and recover more rapidly when challenged by stressors.

10. The above observations on the NRC report on meditation are based on D. W. Orme-Johnson and C. N. Alexander, "Critique of the National Research Council's Report on Meditation." Manuscript available from first author, Department of Psychology, MIU, Fairfield, Iowa 52557-1034.

11. D. L. Radin and R. D. Nelson, "Consciousness-Related Effects in Random Physical Systems," *Foundations of Physics* 19 (1989): 1499–1514.

12. R. S. Broughton, *Parapsychology: The Controversial Science* (New York: Ballantine Books, 1991), 291.

13. C. Honorton and D. C. Ferrari, " 'Future Telling': A Meta-analysis of Forced-choice Precognition Experiments, 1935–1987," *Journal of Parapsychology* 53 (1989): 281–308.

14. Broughton, *Parapsychology: The Controversial Science*, 323–24.

APPENDIX 4. HEALING AND THE MIND:
A SUMMING UP

1. Jeffrey S. Levin, "Esoteric v. Exoteric Explanations for Findings Linking Spirituality and Health," personal communication, June 21, 1993; also to appear in *Advances: The Journal of Mind-Body Health*, in press. Also, Jeffrey S. Levin, *Religion in Aging and Health: Theoretical Foundations and Methodological Frontiers* (Los Angeles: Sage Publications, 1993).

2. J.S. Levin and H.Y. Vanderpool, "Is Frequent Religious Attendance *Really* Conducive to Better Health? Toward an Epidemiology of Religion," *Social Science and Medicine* 24, 1987, 589–600.

3. J.S. Levin, "Religion and Health: Is There an Association, Is it Valid and Is it Causal," *Social Science and Medicine*, in press. Also, J.S. Levin and P.L. Schiller, "Is There a Religious Factor in Health?" *Journal of Religion and Health* 26, 1987, 9–36.

4. J. S. Levin, "Esoteric v. Exoteric Explanations for Findings Linking Spiritu-

ality and Health," personal communication, June 21, 1993; also to appear in *Advances: The Journal of Mind-Body Health*, in press.

5. D.B. Larson and S.S. Larson, "Religious Commitment and Health: Valuing the Relationship," Second Opinion: Health, Faith, and Ethics 17:1, 1991, 26-40. Larson and Larson have assembled a teaching module which physicians could fruitfully follow in dealing with the delicate issues of spirituality and religious practices with patients, without appearing to be an advocate of any particular religious tradition or point of view: "The Forgotten Factor in Physical and Mental Health: Want Does the Research Show? An Independent Study Seminar" (Washington, D.C.: National Institute for Healthcare Research, 1992). Interestingly, those physicians who were not religious seemed to achieve better results at inquiry than physicians who were.

6. F.C. Craigie, Jr., D.B. Larson, and I.Y. Liu, "References to Religion in *The Journal of Family Practice:* Dimensions and Valence of Spirituality," *The Journal of Family Practice* 30:4, 1990, 477-80.

Index

(Italic page references indicate tables.)

Permissions

Grateful acknowledgment is made to the following for permission to reprint material:

Advances: The Journal of Mind/Body Health, from David Spiegel, "A Psychosocial Intervention and Survival Time of Patients with Metastatic Breast Cancer," vol. 7, no. 3, © 1991, The Fetzer Institute, Kalamazoo, MI.

Anchor Books, from Nick Herbert, *Quantum Reality*, © 1987, Anchor Books/Bantam Doubleday Dell Publishing Group, Inc., New York, NY.

Ballantine Books/Random House, Inc., from Richard Broughton, *Parapsychology: The Controversial Science*, © 1991, Ballantine Books/Random House, Inc., New York, NY.

Bantam Books, from Ernest Kurtz and Katherine Ketcham, *The Spirituality of Imperfection*, © 1992, Bantam Books/Bantam Doubleday Dell Publishing Group, Inc., New York, NY.

William G. Braud, from "The Influence of Consciousness in the Physical World: A Psychologist's View," paper presented to the Second International Symposium on Science and Consciousness, Athens, Greece, January 3–7, 1992; from "Healing Analog Research and Human Consciousness," paper presented at the Annual Meeting of the Society for the Scientific Study of Religion and the Religious Research Association, Virginia Beach, VA, November 9–11, 1990; and from "Human Interconnectedness: Research Indications," *ReVision* (1992) vol. 14, no. 3, 140–148, © 1992 by Helen Dwight Reid Educational Foundation.

Cambridge University Press, from Paul Davies, *Space and Time in the Modern Universe*, © 1977, Cambridge University Press, North American Branch, New York, NY.

DeVorss & Co., from Max Freedom Long, *The Secret Science Behind Miracles: Unveiling the Huna Tradition of the Ancient Polynesians*, © 1976, DeVorss & Co., Marina Del Rey, CA.

Dutton Signet/Penguin USA, from L. L. Vasiliev, *Experiments in Distant Influence*, Anita Gregory, trans., © 1963 by the Institute for the Study of Mental Images under the title *Experiments in Mental Suggestion*. Introduction © 1976 by Anita Gregory, Dutton Signet/Penguin USA, Inc., New York, NY.

289

Dennis Gersten, M.D., editor, for "Interview with Janet Quinn, R.N., Ph.D., 'AIDS, Hope and Healing,' Part II," *Atlantis: The Imagery Newsletter,* 4016 Third Avenue, San Diego, CA. February, 1992, pp. 3ff.

HarperCollins Publishers Inc., from Richard J. Foster, *Prayer: Finding the Heart's True Home,* © 1992 by Richard Foster. Also from Jayne Gackenbach and Jane Bosveld, *Control Your Dreams,* © 1989; also from Aldous Huxley, *The Perennial Philosophy,* © 1944; also from Abraham M. Maslow, *The Psychology of Science,* © 1966. HarperCollins Publishers Inc., New York, NY. Reprinted by permission of Harper-Collins Publishers, Inc.

Helix Verlag GmbH, from Daniel J. Benor, *Healing Research,* © 1993, Helix Verlag GmbH, Windeckstr. 82, D–81375 Munich, Germany.

Institute of Noetic Sciences, from Willis W. Harman, *A Reexamination of the Metaphysical Foundations of Modern Science,* © 1991, Institute of Noetic Sciences, 475 Gate Five Road, Suite 300, Sausalito, CA.

Journal of Scientific Exploration, for Robert G. Jahn, Brenda J. Dunne, and Roger D. Nelson, "Engineering Anomalies Research," vol. 1, no. 1, pp. 21–50, © 1987, *Journal of Scientific Exploration,* ERL 306, Stanford University, Stanford, CA.

Little, Brown and Company, from Larry Berger, Dahlia Lithwick, and Seven Campers, *I Will Sing Life: Voices from the Hole in the Wall Gang Camp,* © 1992, Little Brown and Company, Boston, MA.

MacMillan Publishing Company, from Sir James G. Frazer, *The Golden Bough,* © 1992, Macmillan Publishing Company, New York, NY.

McFarland & Company, Inc., from Jerry Solfvin, "Mental Healing," in *Advances in Parapsychological Research 4,* Stanley Krippner, editor, ©1984, McFarland & Co., Inc., Publishers, Jefferson, NC.

National Geographic, from Will Steger, "Six Across Antarctica," © National Geographic Society, Washington, D.C.

Pantheon Books, from Carl G. Jung, *Memories, Dreams, Reflections,* © 1965, Vintage Books, New York, NY.

Parabola, from "ARCS: The Dance of Healing," vol. XVIII, no. 1, © 1993, *Parabola,* New York, NY.

Penguin Books Ltd., from Clifton Wolters, trans., *The Cloud of Unknowing and Other Works,* © 1964, London, UK.

Princeton University Press, from *Jung's Letters,* vol. 1, Gerhard Adler and Aniela Jaffe ©, editors, © 1973, Princeton University Press, Princeton, NJ.

Random House, Inc., from Ralph Waldo Emerson, "The Over-Soul," in *Essays: First and Second Series,* © 1990, First Vintage Books/The Library of America Edition, Random House, Inc., New York, NY.

Shambhala Publications, Inc., from Holger Kalweit, *Shamans, Healers, and Medicine Men,* © 1992, Shambhala Publications, Inc., Boston, MA.

Jeremy P. Tarcher, Inc., from Michael Murphy, *The Future of the Body,* © 1992, Jeremy P. Tarcher, Inc., Los Angeles, CA.

Author's Request

My research in prayer continues. I would appreciate hearing from readers who would be willing to share their experiences. I am especially interested in five areas: "hopeless" situations in which ordinary medical interventions failed but in which prayer seemed to work, time-displaced prayer, negative prayer effects, prayer involving dreams, and telesomatic events. Please write to me at the following address:

Larry Dossey, M.D.
223 N. Guadalupe, #169
Santa Fe, NM 87501

Thank you.